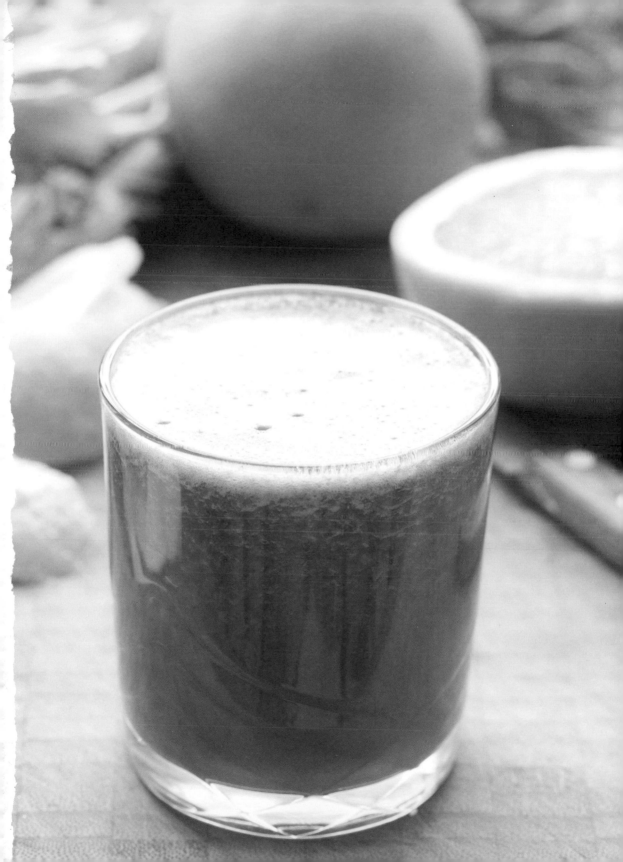

PRAISE FOR
THE ALKALINE CURE BOOK

'Glow like Gwyneth with recipes from Dr. Stephen Domenig, head medical doctor at top detox destination for the rich and famous.'
Alexia Dellner, *Women's Health*

'Learn how to balance the body's pH by trading acidic foods, which lead to fat and fatigue, for alkaline foods, which heal the body.'
Melissa Sorrells, *Closer Weekly*

'The Alkaline Cure is not just a "diet" but an approach to eating, including manners and awareness, as well as achieving a balance in your atmosphere and environment – not just food.'
Lucy Walton, *Female First*

'It shows you how to prepare yourself and your shelves for the best possible plan results … to leave you lighter, brighter and with bucketloads more energy in just a matter of days.'
Emma Jones, *Get the Gloss*

'A miracle cure, based on the diagnostic principles of Dr F. X. Mayr … I arrived home several kilograms lighter with glowing skin and a renewed sense of vitality.'
Charlene Barton, *Matches Fashion*

'It is not a fad or an extreme diet. It is a book written on well founded principles by a medical practitioner with lots of experience … '
Susan Thira, *Happy Healthy Mumma*

PRAISE FOR
THE ALKALINE APPROACH

'It can heal a wide range of ailments including arthritis, diabetes and cancer, as well as slowing the ageing process ... can improve energy levels and memory and help prevent headaches, bloating, heart disease, muscle pain and insomnia.'
Kate Hilpern, *Independent*

'Finding our way back to equilibrium [through an alkaline diet] is a great chance to improve overall health.'
Hilary Boddie, *European Spa Magazine*

'The alkaline diet has been around for more than a century ... it can help anything from headaches to heart disease.'
Patrick Strudwick, *Mail Online*

'You lose so much without doing anything extreme. I love it!'
Woman's World

'Alkaline foods are easier for the digestive system to break down and therefore vitamins and minerals are more easily absorbed.'
Suzannah Ramsdale, *Marie Claire*

'The diet, the chewing, the massages and the emphasis on drinking water all contribute to my feeling much better ... I rarely feel hungry – evidence, if it were needed, that I routinely eat too much'
Harriet Green, *The Guardian*

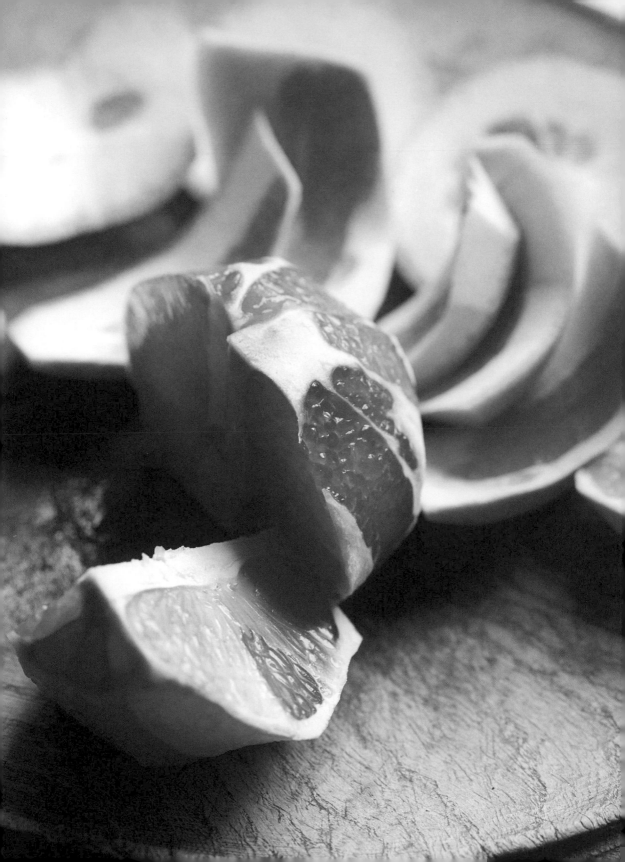

the Alkaline Cleanse

a seven-day detox

DR STEPHAN DOMENIG

with MARTYNA ANGELL

FX MAYR HEALTH CENTER *The Original*

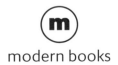

modern books

CONTENTS

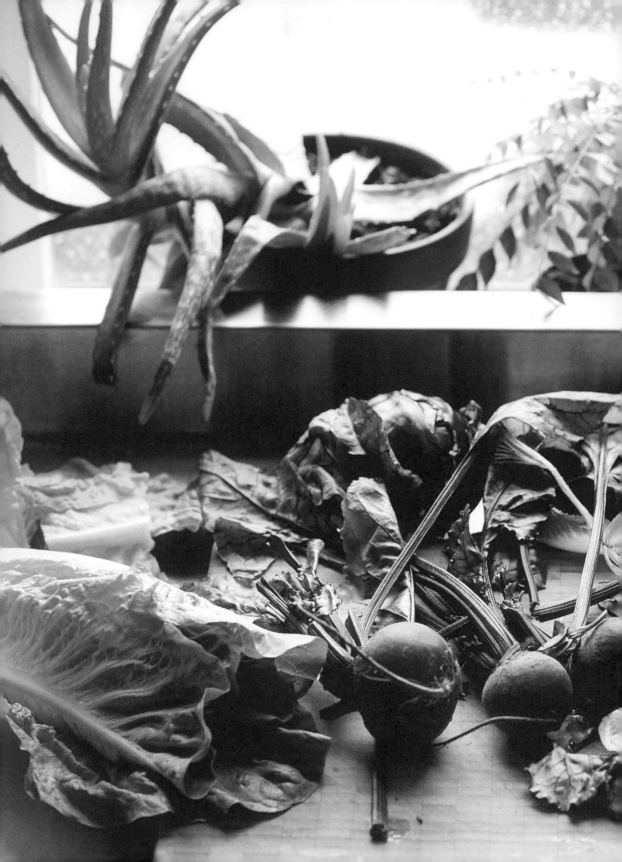

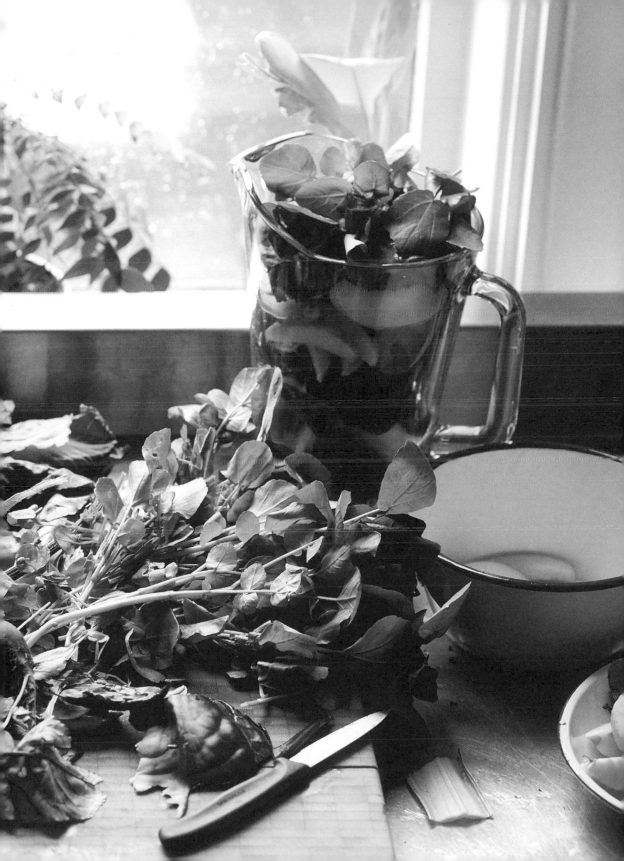

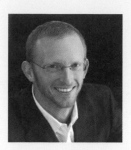

Dr Stephan Domenig
Medical Director
The FX Mayr
Health Center,
Lake Wörthersee,
Austria

At the FX Mayr Health Center on Lake Wörthersee in Austria, we see nearly 100 patients a week. Over 40 years we have accumulated massive amounts of evidence from real patients demonstrating that our holistic approach to cleansing the body is physiologically therapeutic. Numerous research studies have established that the kind of diet most of us eat is a major cause of many illnesses.

Although the benefits of juicing have been known for most of the 20th century, the technology has not really been available to make the idea mainstream. Mayr himself obviously did not include juices in his dietary approach – originally he advocated raw, unpasteurized milk – but here we have taken his principles and applied them to what can be achieved using modern technology. In Ayurvedic thinking everyone should have a liquid fast at least once a week. In that sense juicing is not new but thousands of years old – just the technology makes it easier and more interesting.

Some fruits that may seem to be acid – lime, lemon, grapefruit – in fact have an alkalising effect on the body. Strange but true. But also, if you are going to include any acidic foods in your diet, then the start of the day is the best time. If you eat raw foods in the evening then they will ferment in the stomach overnight because the body just won't have the time to digest them overnight. Like you, your body sleeps too. Raw foods need to be eaten early in the day when your body is strong and has time to absorb their benefits.

In the plan you may find you do not eat as much as you have been doing – which is a good thing because nearly all of us eat too much. But what you do drink is of very high nutritional quality. Plus, hydrating with smoothies, teas, soup and water will help to clean your body. We eat too much acidic food because we like it, after all. The recipes here will help to you to change your mind and see that alkaline foods can be just as delicious and more rewarding.

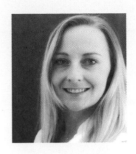

Martyna Angell
Health Coach with the
Institute for Integrative
Nutrition and creator of the
Wholesome Cook blog

I wanted to get involved with *The Alkaline Cleanse* to highlight an important fact: we, as consumers, have the choice to vote with our food spend every time we go shopping. I believe that the food we eat should not only be good for us, but that it should be real. It should be grown and harvested in a way that's responsible to our environment and in a way that shows respect and care for the thing that it is.

Smoothies, juices and plant-based soups made with organic, pesticide-free ingredients are a prime example of food that nourishes. They are a pleasure to drink and are one of the easiest ways to enjoy additional servings of fruit, vegetables, nuts and seeds in our diets. Things that, let's be honest, most of us don't eat enough of in today's world of over-processed and pre-packaged food. Most take less than a few minutes to make and can be enjoyed on the go, transported easily and, in many cases, stored in the fridge for up to 12 hours which means they are as easily accessible as a convenient snack.

The Seven Day Cleanse gives us a chance to reboot our systems and clear out the junk in our diets and our bodies. However, you don't need to cleanse for the whole seven days. One day a week, or a few consecutive days can be enough to get the vital, gut-cleansing nutrition we need into our lives.

In my work as a health coach, recipe developer and food writer I try to create a point of reference for healthy, nutritious and easy-to-prepare meals. I like to think of it as an anti-revolution to the world of highly processed and pre-packaged meals. A way of thinking very similar to that of Dr Stephan Domenig's and his team. And, in the same way, I encourage my readers to nourish their bodies simply with real food.

I hope that the following information, notes and recipes will help you find your own path to healthy living.

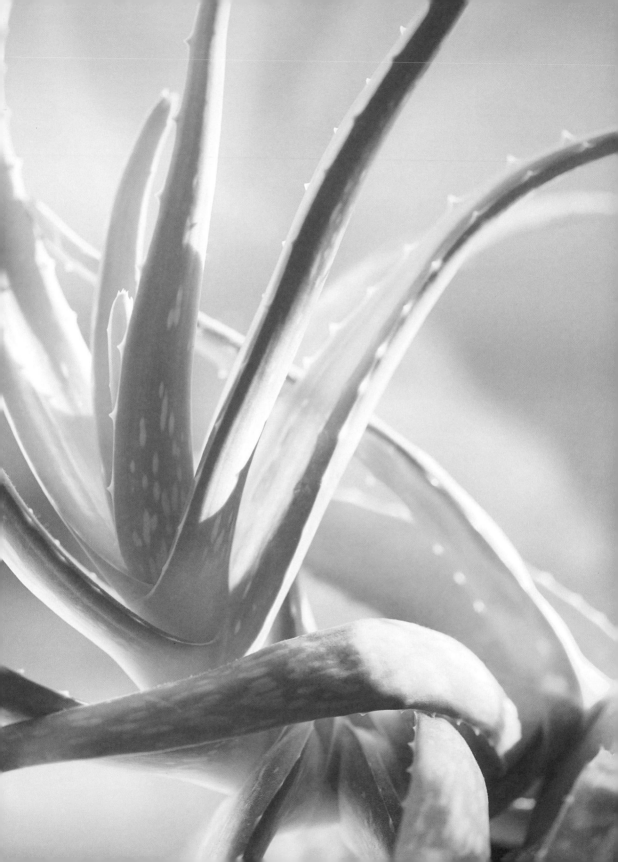

1
Why Alkaline?

What is the Alkaline Cleanse?

Principles of an Alkaline Diet

Mindfulness During the Cleanse

Move your Body

Amazing Benefits of the Alkaline Cleanse

Reasons to Start the Cleanse Now

How Smoothies and Juices Cleanse

Juice or Smoothie?

Ingredients for your Alkaline Cleanse

Can you Juice It?

Teas and Tisanes

Broths and Soups

WHAT IS THE ALKALINE CLEANSE?

A healthy diet means eating a balance of acid and alkaline foods. The modern Western diet is heavily weighted towards foods that we would define as acid-forming. *The Alkaline Cleanse* gives you an easy-to-follow way to cleanse your system and repair that imbalance.

In the Mayr philosophy, the most important route to good health is to support your stomach. If you eat the right things in the right way then your body can cleanse itself. You may want to lose some weight, but alkaline eating is not simply a weight-loss approach; it is a plan for vitality. We are looking for your body to return to its natural shape so it functions at its optimum.

Why a Seven-Day Cleanse?
The Seven-Day Cleanse (see pages 48–93) is designed to be a cleansing fix, providing nutritionally balanced juices, smoothies and soups that will restore and revive your digestive system in a week. Most people do not eat the amount of vegetables and fruit that is recommended (five to seven portions a day), or get the vitamins, minerals and fibre their bodies need. The Seven-Day Cleanse is a quick way to get these into your diet – your body will thank you.

You can follow the plan for seven consecutive days or spread the plan out and do, say, one day a week. You can also skip around the recipes and grab a few nourishing drinks when you feel like a health boost. Use them to top up your alkalising intake and re-engineer what you eat. Even if you only eat alkaline just a couple of days a week, you will experience the benefits.

HOW ACIDIC ARE YOU?

You can test to see how acid or alkaline you are with pH strips that you can buy online and in many health food shops. Just put a little saliva on a strip and see what colour it turns. You want to be in the middle of the colour scale – just over 7pH – which is just leaning towards alkaline. If your reading is below 7pH than you need to adjust your acid levels by following an alkaline plan.

Why do I need to juice?

Making juices and soups at home is so much better than buying imitations on the high street. You control the nutrition – you won't get drinks with added salt, sugar and less fibre. Home-made is fresher, so all the nutrients and vitamins are at their peak. Thanks to technological advances in juice machines we can also now extract the goodness from ingredients in ways which were impossible a few years ago. As a result, making your own juices is fast and easy, and from a digestive point of view they are also super-rich and nutritious.

Your stomach needs time to absorb all the goodness; there is no point filling up with more than your digestive system is able to deal with. A well-balanced juice should be like a glass of wine – something to sip slowly and to appreciate for what it is, the fruit of the earth.

One word of caution: juices can be intense for your digestion. We have become accustomed to thinking that fruit juices should be thick and strong, but in fact many of them taste a lot better if they are diluted, as in the recipes in this book. The occasional thick juice shot is OK, but otherwise dilute your juices. Adding plenty of water to your diet is essential for your digestion.

We do not recommend raw juices or smoothies in the evening as they are too much for your body to digest at this time. Raw food is strictly a daytime thing. Drink teas, tisanes and infusions in the evenings and, if you need something more substantial, home-made soup. These contain many of the same nutritional benefits as juices, but are much easier for the body to absorb.

How often should I cleanse?

Ancient Ayurvedic teaching suggests that everyone should have a liquid fast for one day, every week. Other diets suggest two days a week. If you really want to lose weight, then you can cleanse for the full seven days.

There is more than enough nutrition to keep you going for a whole week in the Seven-Day Cleanse, or you can just use it as a guide for one day each week for seven weeks. Or mix-and-match to suit you; do what makes you feel happiest.

PRINCIPLES OF AN ALKALINE DIET

The Alkaline Cleanse follows the teachings of the Austrian physician Dr FX Mayr who first advocated a set of alkaline dietary and lifestyle principles nearly 100 years ago. These simple principles are still followed at the FX Mayr Health Center on Lake Wörthersee, Austria, and were set out in the first book created with the clinic, *The Alkaline Cure*. In *The Alkaline Cleanse*, we build on these principles to show you how an alkaline way of life can be fast-tracked through a healthy plant-based cleanse.

For Dr Mayr, the stomach was the most important organ in the body. If we look after our stomachs then many of the common ailments that we take for granted such as poor skin, bad breath, excessive gas and constipation start to disappear. Conditions and diseases such as arthritis, Type 2 diabetes and even cancer can respond to an alkaline diet.

There are key principles of the FX Mayr alkaline diet that you can follow to get the most from your cleanse:

* Drink two litres of water each day – this can include your juice content, but there should be plenty of water too. Don't stop drinking water and start drinking only carrot juice instead, for example. Drinking two litres a day helps to keep your core and its organs supple and pliant.

* If you feel hungry between meals drink some Vegetable Tea (see page 57) or filtered water. Sometimes our bodies are thirsty rather than hungry and it is better to drink than eat.

* Don't drink or eat raw food in the evening because it is hard to digest. The food can ferment in your stomach during the night.

* Drink juice, herb tea and soup instead of black tea or coffee. Black tea and coffee are acidic.

* Don't stress yourself over *The Alkaline Cleanse*; stay calm and mindful. Enjoy the process of cleansing your body and spirit.

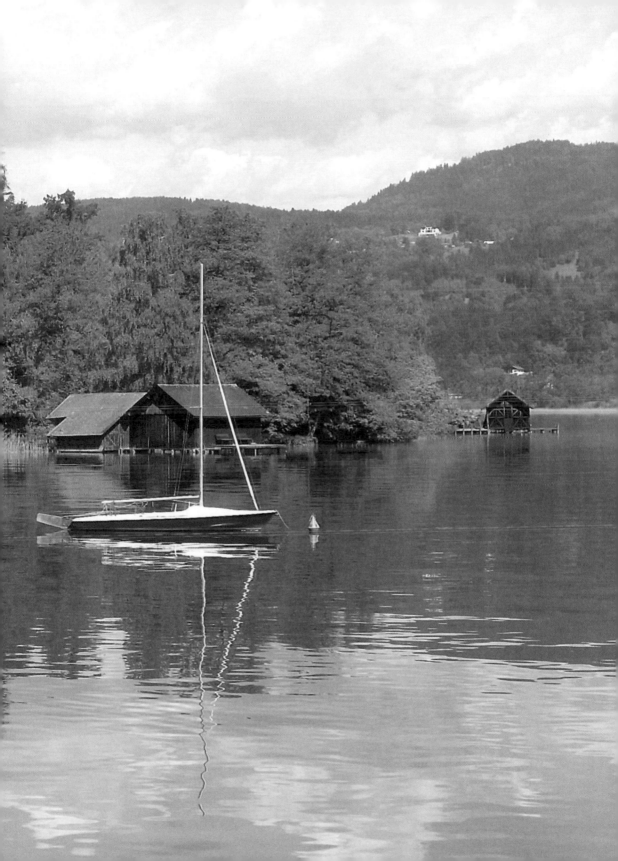

MINDFULNESS DURING THE CLEANSE

When you meditate you try to clear your mind of all the clutter that has managed to find a home for itself. *The Alkaline Cleanse* should work in the same way for your body. If you have been eating anything like a typical Western diet then you will have built up toxins, overloaded your liver and kidneys, and created fat blockages in your colon. It's time for this to change.

Aim for a calm, measured and mindful approach. You know how people can buy a coffee and sit in a coffee shop sipping it for half an hour? You are going to have that approach to enjoying your juices, teas and soups. Sit down and make time for it. This is your time to relax and savour the delicious and healthy food you have made for yourself.

* Give feeding yourself pride of place in your priorities. That little juice you just whizzed up is keeping you alive. Respect it. It is going to make you feel better. Give it a chance.

* Set a time in your mind for breakfast, lunch and dinner. Try to stick with them. This helps you to plan ahead and also tells your body when to expect food.

* Display your beautiful fruit and vegetables in the kitchen. Bunches of fresh herbs, piles of perfect vegetables and fruits look appetising and can inspire unusual combinations.

* Arrange your breakfast vegetables and fruits on a plate the night before so your first meal of the day is easy to prepare.

* Choose a nice glass or cup to serve your drink – one that matches the drink and enhances its appeal. Use your favourite soup bowl.

* Make the preparation enjoyable. You might want to buy a new chopping board and a new sharp knife. Wash and tidy up as you go along so there is no mess and stress later.

* Keep at it. You cannot expect one glass of juice to change your life but making these recipes a regular part of your diet will.

MOVE YOUR BODY

Diet is only half the equation. You can follow the recipes here, yet if you sit on the sofa all day or in a car they won't make the difference you want; your body has to move. Exercise is the key. You don't have to take up bodybuilding but you do have to move around and occasionally work up a sweat.

In the Mayr philosophy we do not believe that you have to be a great athlete to get great health benefits – some of us are naturally more athletic than others – a 30-minute walk in fresh air three or four times a week will help to keep your body and stomach toned and functioning well.

The most important exercise for good digestion is anything that moves the torso. If you do not move the essential organs of the core – the liver, kidneys, stomach and colon – they start to solidify and change your body shape. In the clinic we set a lot of importance on abdominal massage which helps to move the organs so they are free of obstructions and can function freely.

Some form of stomach twisting exercise is worthwhile every day and will bring many of the same benefits as a massage. Twisting or rotating the core allows the organs to re-align and find their natural space. Many routines in the gym tend to be vertical in that they strengthen your thighs, hips and shoulders. Yoga exercises that involve stretching and turning the stomach will also be beneficial.

TWIST AND TURN YOUR BODY

Stand with your feet apart and swing your arms slowly sideways so your body turns around as far as it will go, so you look over your shoulder. Return to face forward and swing around to the other side. Repeat 20 times to each side, making the movement more fluid as you get used to it.

AMAZING BENEFITS OF THE ALKALINE CLEANSE

The good news about an alkaline diet is that the body responds quickly. Within a few days the benefits will start to be obvious. In fact, most of our body renews itself over three months so the longer you carry on the healthier and more vital you will feel. In just seven days you will start to feel and see the benefits of an alkaline diet. Your body will thank you for it.

1. YOU WILL GET THE NUTRIENTS YOUR BODY NEEDS

Packed with minerals and vitamins, you will consume a variety of vegetables, fruits and herbs, each with their own mix of nutrients.

2. YOU CAN LOSE WEIGHT

The juices, smoothies, soups and teas contain all the nutrients you need. If you stick to the plan you will be surprised at how much weight you can lose, even in just seven days.

3. YOUR BODY WILL DETOX

Over time the body builds up toxins. If you are eating a poor diet, one of the side effects is the body gets lazy and does not clean itself. The fibre in the recipes will wash all that away.

4. YOU WILL LOOK BETTER

Your friends will notice, perhaps before you, the effect of the cleanse. The whites of your eyes will be whiter. Your skin will glow. That is because we are getting rid of all the toxins your body has accumulated.

5. YOU WILL FEEL BETTER

The recipes are easy to digest and are packed with the nutrition you need. Eating vegetables, fruit and herbs in liquid form is the easiest way to ensure your body is able to absorb the goodness and can get what it needs, when it needs it.

6. YOU WILL PERFORM BETTER

As your body is getting what it needs, your mind and body will be able to function better; you will be able to think more clearly, and will feel more energetic and agile. Your bowel movements will become easy and you won't be susceptible to uncomfortable bloating or gas.

7. YOU WILL BE HAPPILY HYDRATED

Most of us do not drink nearly as much as we need. Two litres of water a day is a minimum – three would be ideal. Drinking what your body needs tones your muscles and makes your joints flexible. It also washes out your kidneys.

8. YOU WILL ENJOY THE RECIPES

The recipes taste good; they are delicious and varied so you will want to try them and stick with them.

9. THE PLAN IS EASY

There is nothing in this book that takes a long time to prepare, and you may find you save time compared to your usual cooking. The juices and smoothies only take a minute or two to prepare and even our soups don't take long; we cook for a short time to retain their vitamins and minerals. *The Alkaline Cleanse* can fit into your life.

10. IT MIGHT JUST CHANGE YOUR LIFE

Trying something new is good for the soul; discovering a new way to eat that makes you feel great is exciting!

REASONS TO START
THE CLEANSE NOW

Modern juicers are fast, efficient and easy to clean, whereas only a few years ago they were cumbersome and messy. They would sit in the corner of the kitchen brooding and unused for a while before finding their rightful homes being sold online or at a car boot sale.

Juicing has got easier

The first juicer was only invented in 1936 by a raw food enthusiast, Norman Wardhaugh Walker, who opened the world's first juice bar on Long Beach, California. His machine, the Norwalk, was cumbersome and labour-intensive using two processes – first grinding the ingredients and then pressing them to squeeze out the juice. Now, juicers and blenders and quick and easy to use, providing us with an easy path to increased nutrition.

It can make mealtimes easier

From your stomach's point of view a glassful of orange juice is an overload. Would you ever eat as many whole oranges as go in one glass? Of course not. Balance is the key – a balanced body, balanced mind. Dr Walker labelled all his first juicers with the motto: 'Eat your fruit and juice your veg' to warn people that it is far too easy to consume too much sugary fruit juice in one go.

LOOKING AFTER YOUR PANCREAS

Your pancreas plays a crucial part in good digestion. The pancreas neutralises the acid in your stomach and helps break down the food you eat. It also produces insulin which reduces your blood sugar levels and helps the body store energy. A few foods are especially helpful to the pancreas including blueberries, cherries, broccoli, cauliflower, cabbage and Brussels sprouts. Kitchen staples garlic and onions are great too; it is no coincidence that nearly every soup recipe you will ever read starts with onions – there is an old wisdom to it.

Rather than a sugar-hit, think of your smoothie as a balanced meal – containing vegetables, fibre, herbs, spices and healthy fats from nuts or oils. Remember though, fruit becomes alkaline only as it ripens. A lot of supermarkets sell unripe fruit so you will need to let it ripen before you use it. Superfoods that target and boost the performance of every organ in the body will also be a part of your week becoming alkaline.

Juicing is fast and convenient. In the morning, you can mix in your favourite breakfast staples like oats or muesli-style mixes, even yogurts. Rather than a protein-heavy meal loaded with fats and carbohydrates, a fibre-rich smoothie takes minutes to prepare and will contain all the alkaline ingredients you need for breakfast or lunch. Likewise, a nourishing soup can be thrown together in a matter of moments and will happily steep for a few days afterwards so that you always have a substantial, gut-pleasing dinner on hand.

It is affordable

It is also cheap to go alkaline. Apart from a little technology to help with the more daunting tasks, all you need is a supply of fresh fruits, vegetables and greens. Even buying the variety we suggest will cost you less than your usual shopping. If you like to plan ahead and have a freezer you can save money by buying in bulk. Many juice books recommend using frozen ingredients for convenience but fresh is ideal for speed and handling; unpacking a bag of frozen fruit does not quite feel as sensual as unzipping a banana. That said, freezing is a great way to make sure nothing is wasted, and a few frozen berries can make a pretty garnish.

You will feel better, very quickly

Readjusting your diet to an alkaline perspective is going to make you feel better quickly. A week of balanced eating and drinking will allow a digestive system that has spent too long trying to battle against what it receives to rest and heal. This, combined with increased liquid intake and some gentle exercise, is the fast path to a healthier lifestyle.

HOW SMOOTHIES
AND JUICES CLEANSE

The Alkaline Cleanse contains a wide range of alkaline foods that combine to have a fast, cleansing, detoxing effect on your body. Absolutely everything in this cleanse is alkaline, and each ingredient will do you good. Each juice, smoothie, soup and porridge will work its way around your eight metres of gut and colon, repairing them and flushing out the toxins that a sedentary, protein-rich lifestyle will have created. That is quite a long way to have to clean, so it may take a few days.

Some recipes will have a greater effect than others on your body, depending on what they encounter, so listen to your body. Boosting ingredients such as flax, spirulina, spices and oils can be easily included in smoothies and juices too, and this will help to add even more benefits to the fruits and vegetables you will be consuming every day. Flaxseed oil is a rare source of omega 3 although many people don't like the taste, but you could grind the seeds instead. The most important thing is to enjoy what you are doing, and stay focused on your own body. It is an alkaline lifestyle that we are aiming for, so if you don't like something, don't get hung up about it.

A NOTE ON ALLERGIES

One by-product of a modern western diet is we develop intolerances to certain foods – milk for example, the gluten in bread, histamine in aged cheeses and old wines. Essentially what is happening is our bodies can only consume so much and we reach a tipping point where we have maxed out or just run out of tolerance. The body gets angry and fights back. *The Alkaline Cleanse* cuts out almost all of these foods, providing your body with the natural goodness it craves. You are the best judge of your body. You are its best doctor. Sit your stomach down in your surgery and listen to what it has to say.

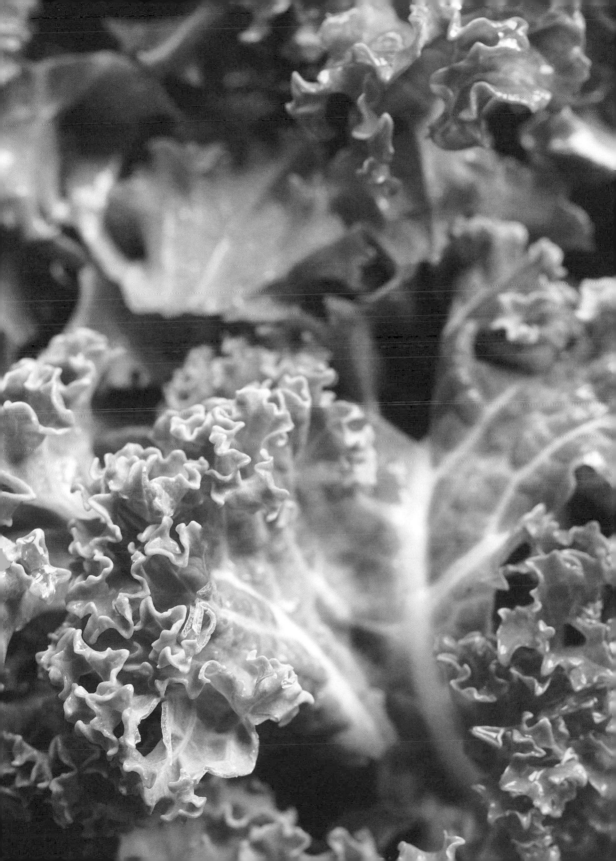

JUICE OR SMOOTHIE?

We include recipes for juices and smoothies in the cleanse and both are useful in your diet.

Juicing extracts the juice from the fruit or vegetable, leaving the fibrous parts behind. Juicing machines have really developed in recent years; they can now extract more juice from your ingredients – even such unlikely-looking vegetables as beetroot – or squeeze out the essence from a leaf of spinach, kale or wheatgrass. How much juice you extract depends on the capability of your machine – not all machines can juice everything (see page 44).

In a juice you get all the vitamins, minerals and flavours of your ingredients, but no fibre. Minerals and vitamins disappear when exposed to oxygen so a good juice is made to order by you and is best drunk immediately. You are less likely to chew while drinking a juice, which means you bypass an important part of the digestive process. The saliva you generate when eating is an important part of your chemistry, so make sure you drink slowly.

You can juice raw vegetables to add to drinks and soups; adding to soup is a clever way of speeding the preparation and getting the best colour and nutrition into the dish.

Smoothies are made in a blender by whizzing whole fruits and vegetables together which means you keep all the fibre in the drink. You can thicken them with grains such as oats, creamy banana or avocado. You can also add nutrient-rich ingredients that you are not sure you are going to like; pop in a few seeds or some spirulina and whizz away. Make sure you have enough liquid in there so nuts and seeds break down well. Because smoothies contain fibre they are better than juices at sweeping bad things out of your colon. You want your smoothie smooth but not warm, so the moment the machine starts to heat up, turn it off.

Smoothies are probably best taken early in the day for breakfast so the body has plenty of time to absorb all the fibre and goodness. Juices are ideal used as power shots later in the day. You can also use juice as part of a smoothie and get the best of both worlds.

INGREDIENTS FOR YOUR ALKALINE CLEANSE

GREEN VEGETABLES

Granny would tell you to eat your greens, but we say drink them. Green plants provide amino acids that are the building blocks of protein, in a way that is much easier for the body to absorb than meat and dairy.

GREEN VEGETABLE	NUTRIENTS	GREEN VEGETABLE	NUTRIENTS
All herbs	Herbs contain countless beneficial nutrients – use widely	Fennel	Vitamin C, potassium, molybdenum, manganese, copper
Avocado	Pantothenic acid, vitamin K, copper, folate, vitamin B6	Kale	Vitamin K, vitamin A, vitamin C, manganese, copper
Broccoli	Vitamin K, vitamin C, chromium, folate, vitamin B6	Kohlrabi	Vitamin C, phytochemicals, niacin, vitamin B6, thiamin
Cabbage	Vitamin K, vitamin C, potassium, vitamin B6, manganese	Rocket	Phytochemicals, vitamin A, B-complex vitamins, iron
Celery	Silicon, polysaccharides, vitamin C	Romaine lettuce	Vitamin K, vitamin A, folate, molybdenum, potassium
Chicory	Thiamin, niacin, zinc, vitamin A, vitamin E	Seaweed	Iodine, calcium, magnesium, vitamin C, vitamin B2
Courgette	Vitamin C, vitamin K, riboflavin, vitamin B6, folate	Spinach	Vitamin A, vitamin C, vitamin E, calcium, iron
Cucumber	Vitamin K, vitamin A, copper, potassium, vitamin C	Spring onions	Antioxidants, phytonutrients, vitamin C, vitamin B2
Dandelion	Vitamin A, vitamin C, vitamin E, thiamin, riboflavin	Wheatgrass	Vitamin A, vitamin C, vitamin E, vitamin K, niacin

ROOTS AND OTHER VEGETABLES

Carrots and beetroots (including the leaves if they are fresh) are very useful for juices and smoothies, but they are not the only vegetables that can be used. Aim to use a variety of colours – rich reds and oranges, like ripe peppers, will have anti-oxidising properties. Sweet potato juices well and makes a good change from white potato varieties. Potatoes are very alkalising for soups; some people drink raw potato juice but it is not for everyone.

VEGETABLES	NUTRIENTS
Beetroot	Folate, vitamin C, potassium, phosphorus, magnesium
Carrot	Vitamin A, biotin, vitamin K, potassium, phosphorus
Celeriac	Vitamin K, vitamin C, phosphorous, calcium, iron
Parsnip	Vitamin K, vitamin C, manganese, folate, copper
Potato	Vitamin B6, potassium, phosphorus, vitamin C, copper
Sweet potato	Vitamin A, vitamin C, manganese, copper, vitamin B6
Peppers (red, orange, yellow and green)	Vitamin C, vitamin A, vitamin B6, folate, molybdenum

FRUITS

Fruits are alkaline only when they are properly ripe. Dark blue fruits like plums, blueberries and black grapes have an anti-oxidising effect which is especially good for the kidneys. Tropical fruits are extremely alkalising. Melons are the easiest fruit to digest and when ripe can whizz easily to make a delicious smoothie without any added liquid.

FRUITS	NUTRIENTS	FRUITS	NUTRIENTS
Apple	Vitamin A, vitamin B, vitamin C, vitamin E, vitamin K	Mango	Vitamin A, vitamin C, vitamin B6, potassium, copper
Banana	Vitamin B6, vitamin C, manganese, potassium, biotin	Melon (any variety)	Vitamin C, vitamin A, potassium, folate, vitamin B3
Berries (Blueberries, Cranberries, Strawberries, Raspberries, Gooseberries, Blackberries)	Vitamin K, manganese, vitamin C, copper, potassium	Orange	Vitamin C, folate, vitamin B1, potassium, copper
Coconut	Vitamin B6, vitamin C, potassium, manganese, cytokinins	Papaya	Vitamin C, folate, vitamin A, magnesium, potassium
Grape	Vitamin C, vitamin K, vitamin B2, copper, antioxidants	Passion fruit	Vitamin A, vitamin C, potassium, iron, phosphorus
Grapefruit	Vitamin C, copper, vitamin A, potassium, vitamin B1	Pear	Copper, vitamin C, vitamin K, phytonutrients, folates
Kiwi	Vitamin C, vitamin K, copper, vitamin E, potassium	Pineapple	Vitamin C, manganese, copper, vitamin B1, vitamin B6
Lemon	Vitamin C, folate, phytochemicals, iron, copper	Plum	Vitamin C, vitamin K, copper, potassium, vitamin A
Lime	Vitamin C, folate, phytochemicals, iron, copper	Watermelon	Vitamin C, copper, biotin, potassium, vitamin A

WATER, MILK AND JUICES

Use these liquids in your recipes or drink them (as well as lots of filtered water) throughout the day. All fruit juices benefit from being diluted with water – we suggest you make your own as most commercial juices will have reduced nutritional benefits. Cordials, of course, are full of sugar. Cow and goat milks are marginally acidic so use sparingly. Try using coconut milk or almond milk instead, both of which are alkalising.

LIQUID	NUTRIENTS	LIQUID	NUTRIENTS
Almond milk	Vitamin D, vitamin E, calcium, vitamin A, phosphorus	Herb and green teas	Catechins, theanine, vitamin C, vitamin B2, vitamin E
Aloe vera water	Vitamin C, germanium, calcium, zinc, vitamin E	Lemon juice	Vitamin C, folate, phytochemicals, iron, copper
Apple juice	Vitamin C, antioxidants, vitamin B6, phytonutrients	Mango juice	Vitamin A, vitamin C, vitamin B6, potassium, copper
Beetroot juice	Folate, vitamin C, potassium, phosphorus, magnesium	Orange juice	Vitamin C, folate, vitamin B1, potassium, copper
Carrot juice	Vitamin A, biotin, vitamin K, potassium, phosphorus	Prune juice	Vitamin B6, potassium, manganese, vitamin C, vitamin K
Coconut milk or water	Calcium, iron, potassium, vitamin B3, folate	Rhubarb juice	Vitamin A, vitamin C, vitamin K, calcium
Elderflower water	Triterpenes, antioxidants, bioflavonoids, chlorogenic acids	Tomato juice	Vitamin A, vitamin C, vitamin K, vitamin B-6
Grape juice	Vitamin C, vitamin K, vitamin B2, copper, antioxidants	Vegetable Tea (page 57)	This contains all the benefits of its components
Grapefruit juice	Vitamin C, copper, vitamin A, potassium, vitamin B1		

DELICIOUS EXTRAS

Here are some extras that you can add to your food that are actually going to do you good. To make them easy to absorb, mill the seeds just before adding to your juices, smoothies and porridges. It is also a good idea to soak larger ingredients like almonds for a few hours ahead of time to make them easier to digest. If a recipe calls for one kind of seed or nut, feel free to substitute with another you might have.

BOOSTER	NUTRIENTS	BOOSTER	NUTRIENTS
Almonds	Biotin, vitamin E, manganese, copper, vitamin B2	Hemp seeds	Magnesium, zinc, vitamin E, phytonutrients
Almond oil	Vitamin E, omega 6	Horseradish	Vitamin C, potassium, manganese, iron, copper
Amaranth	Vitamin A, vitamin C, folate, calcium, iron	Linseed	Vitamin B1, manganese, copper, phosphorus, magnesium
Avocado oil	Omega 3, omega 6, omega 9	Oats	Potassium, Phosphorus, magnesium, iron, calcium
Cardamom	Potassium, iron, manganese, calcium, magnesium	Olive oil	Omega 6, Omega 3, vitamin E, vitamin K
Chia seeds/flaxseed	Manganese, calcium, phosphorus, antioxidants, Vitamin B1	Pumpkin oil	Omega 6, omega 9, phosphorus, manganese, zinc
Chilli	Vitamin E, vitamin A, vitamin B6, vitamin K, copper	Pumpkin seeds	Vitamin E, manganese, phosphorus, copper, magnesium, zinc
Garlic	Manganese, vitamin B6, vitamin C, copper, selenium	Sunflower seeds	Vitamin E, copper, vitamin B1, manganese, selenium
Ginger root	Vitamin B6, vitamin B5, potassium, manganese, copper	Spirulina	Potassium, vitamin B6, biotin, zinc, calcium

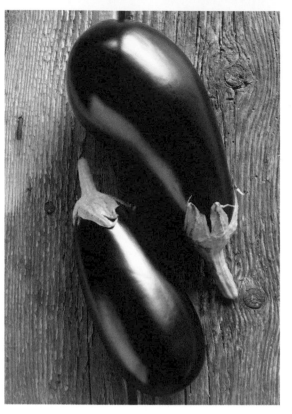

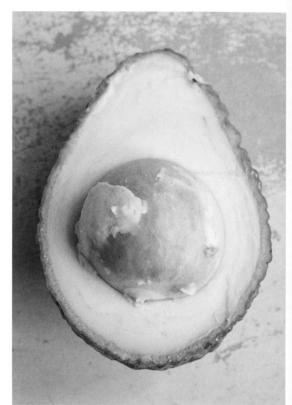

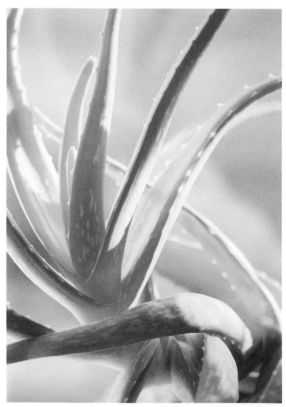

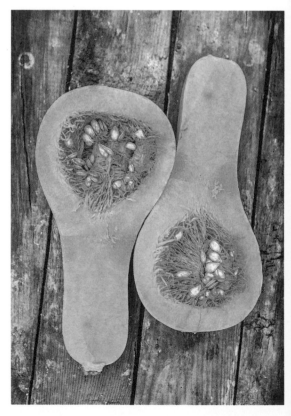

CAN YOU JUICE IT?

Not every fruit and vegetable in the world can be reduced to a satisfactory juice. Some are very good for you and would be useful in an alkaline diet but you will have to handle them in a different way.

Avocados
The creamy texture of an avocado will get stuck in a juicer so you will need to mash it by hand or use a blender with the liquid you are using added. You can also eat them on their own or in a salad, of course.

Bananas
You can blend and mash a banana but it won't like being juiced. Banana oxidises and browns very quickly so be ready to add it to your recipe and drink as soon as possible.

Aloe vera
Always blend aloe vera leaves. If you put them in a juicer there will be some serious cleaning left to do. You can also use aloe vera juice that comes in bottles, but make sure there is no added sugar.

Aubergine
There is just not enough liquid in an aubergine for it to juice effectively. You can bake chunks with a little oil to eat in ratatouille or mash to make a dip.

Leeks
The layers of a leek will jam up a juicing machine and they also have a strong, dominant flavour when raw. They are best cooked and added to soups where you will still get the nutritional benefits. You need to cook leeks only for a short while to soften them.

Squash
A good masticating juicer will be able to process squash and sweet potaoes, but generally they will need to be cooked. They can then be eaten as they are, added to a soup or blended into a smoothie. Summer squashes like courgettes are fine to juice; choose ones with soft skins.

TEAS AND TISANES

Black tea, the one most people drink, is acidic so we don't drink it as part of an alkaline diet. There is also a lot of very expensive rubbish sold as tea in supermarkets. We suggest you make your own tea using fresh and dried herbs, which will be alkaline (see pages 130–137). If you want to buy tea, then green tea is alkaline.

Herbs are often overlooked in the diet, thought of only as flavouring, rather than as a nutritious ingredient in their own right. Herbs were an important part of medicine for centuries until modern drugs took over and we can still enjoy their benefits. You can make a simple herb tea or tisane to be sipped at any time of the day. Essentially, tea is just a herbal or leaf juice.

You can buy fresh herbs quite easily now and of course you can grow your own. Even the smallest garden or window ledge has space for herbs; imagine that the first thing you taste in the morning is hot water with your own mint or sage; it is a special moment.

Almost all herbs make a good tea, and they bring their own range of benefits – some are better for the morning, and others for the evening. If you make extra you can use tea to add a bit of extra character to your smoothies and juices. You can also make teas from various weeds, shrubs and plant roots. Some of the most useful include:

> *aloe vera, basil, borage, burdock, celery, chives, coriander, dandelion, dill, epazote, garlic, ginger, lemongrass, lovage, oregano, parsley, peppermint, rosemary, sage, savory, spearmint, stevia, sweet marjoram, tarragon, thyme, turmeric*

With larger plants like celery or lovage you can make an infusion; leave to steep in boiling water for 10 minutes and then strain. Tough roots such as lemongrass benefit from being pounded first to release their aromatic oils. Most teas benefit from being strained so you can drink the whole tea without ingesting the leaves and fibres; woody herbs impart a bitter flavour if you leave them in water for too long.

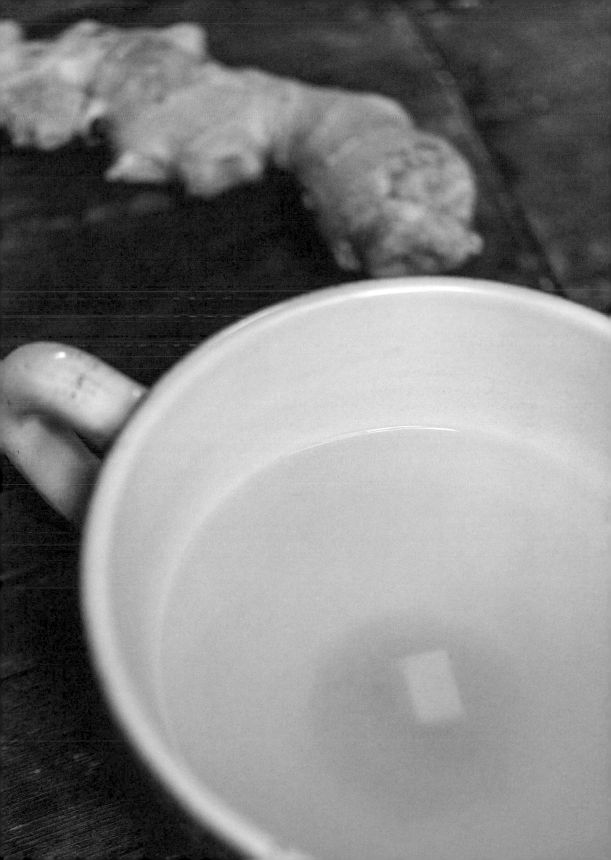

BROTHS AND SOUPS

Broths and soups have sustained our ancestors for generations and we too can benefit from a simple, natural bowl of goodness. A broth tends to be a thinner, more liquid-based soup and is easily sipped from a mug. A soup tends to be thicker, containing more of the cooking vegetables.

During cooking, vegetables are heated and broken down slowly in their cooking water, so the nutrients are that much easier to digest. The cooking process does, in part, what the digestive system has to do. So making soup makes it easy for your body to absorb nutrients and vitamins. You just know that a bowl of home-made soup will do you good. If you want to make sure that you get the recommended amount of vegetables in your day, soup is the easiest way for your stomach to manage it all.

Just throw a variety of vegetables in the pot and off you go. Soup is highly practical because one pot can last for two or three days. If you need to top it up add the water from any vegetables and potatoes that you might be cooking. You can even add leftover juice. The true art of cooking is to make one thing magically transform into something else. So add carrots and parsnips to make vegetable soup, and add leftover potatoes the next day with some broccoli and spinach and the soup is transformed again. The dinner recipes in the Seven-Day Cleanse (see pages 48–93) follow this principle, making cooking quick and easy.

VEGETABLE TEA

Basically a simple broth, you make Vegetable Tea (see page 57) on the first day of the Seven-Day Cleanse and drink it throughout the week. Get into the habit of making this all the time and drink instead of coffee and tea. It is a delicious way to drink more water and it is packed with nutrients. If you make plenty you can use it as stock for your soups and add whatever vegetables you have to make a more substantial meal.

SOUP MADE EASY

Making soup is not time-consuming or difficult – think of it as making a juice in a saucepan, rather than in a juicer. Making soup from your choice of ingredients can be a calming, restorative, restful pleasure in its own right.

Myth 1: You don't have to cook everything in fat first. Lots of recipes start with heating oil then cooking onions. This is not necessary; you can cook everything in water or stock alone. In fact, fat can reduce the nutritional content and make your soup greasy. It is not really necessary.

Myth 2: You don't have to use stock. Water and vegetables can make a delicious soup on their own. If you do want to make a stock it is very easy and won't cost you anything (see below).

Leftovers vegetable stock

The vegetables and greens that you prepare for juicing or soup-making also make a great vegetable stock. Just steal an inch off the bottom of a carrot, the stalks off your kale, a couple of stems of celery or the green tops of spring onion – in fact, a lot of what you juice is going to be useful in the stockpot. Collect up your vegetable leftovers and pop them in a saucepan. Don't worry about precise amounts. Cover with boiling water and simmer for 25 minutes. Strain and there you are – the mysteries of stock-making revealed.

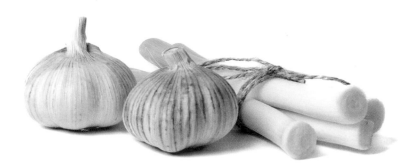

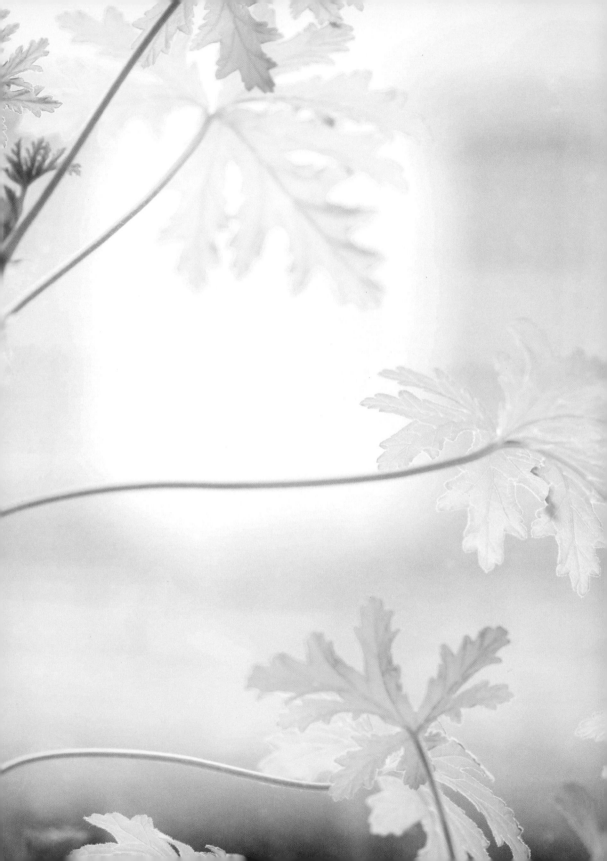

2
Getting Prepared

Shopping and Planning Ahead

Shopping for Ingredients

Shopping List

Choosing Your Equipment

Frequently Asked Questions

SHOPPING AND PLANNING AHEAD

You need a few items of kitchen equipment to do the cleanse, but most of these you will have already. Buying one or two new things can make the cleanse easier and more enjoyable; a new knife or some pretty glasses are not expensive.

If you are doing the Seven-Day Cleanse you might like to treat yourself to a new chopping board; wood or plastic is fine – the boards you can flex to tip ingredients into a blender or saucepan might be useful. Buy a new knife or get your knives sharpened; sharp knives make chopping quicker and safer. You can use the money you are going to save on your old grocery bill.

Use your best glasses; try wine glasses, cocktail glasses and shot glasses. Buy a new, taller glass that can fit in a whole smoothie. Choose something that will make you feel that your meal is an occasion.

An insulated flask is useful to take your juices, smoothies, teas and soups to work with you. You can buy bowl-shaped flasks which are perfect for soup. Think of the money you will save by not buying lunch out each day. Invest in a filter jug too, so you always have water ready to top up smoothies.

Juices are best drunk cold. You can use frozen fruit or keep some fruit in the fridge so it is cold before you use it. Otherwise, an ice cube tray in the freezer will give you enough ice for a day or two.

You will need

juicer or blender (see pages 44–46)	various sizes of drinking glasses
citrus press	soup bowl
large saucepan	cup or mug
chopping board	insulated flask
sharp knife	ice cube tray

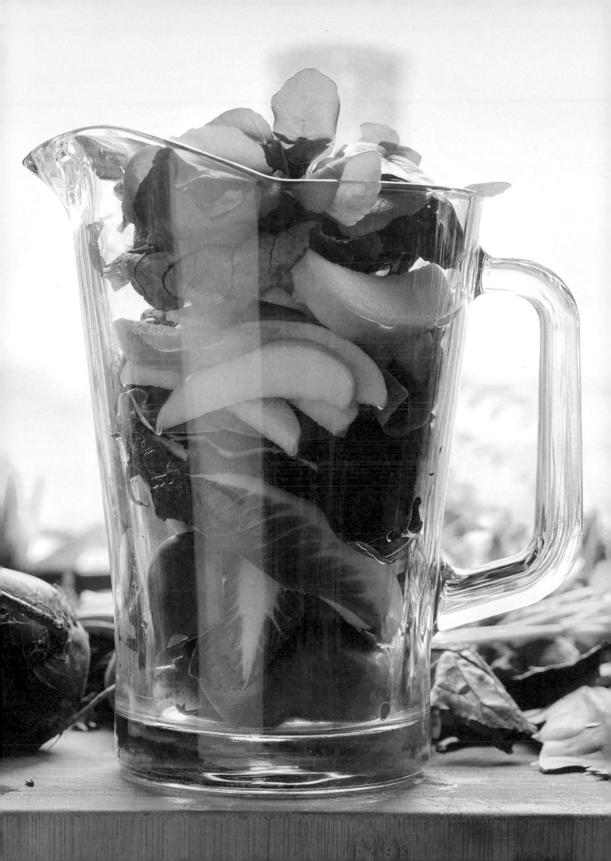

SHOPPING FOR INGREDIENTS

Careful shopping is a part of the cleanse; take time to choose the best-quality fruit and vegetables to give you the best possible flavour and nutrition in your juices, soups and smoothies.

Pick up the fruit and vegetables; feel if they are ripe. Notice how vegetables at their peak are crisp and firm. Make time to go to where your ingredients are grown and visit the local farmers' markets. Choose recipes that make the most of what is in season. Remind yourself of the growing seasons and discover new varieties; some varieties of apples and plums, for example, don't make it into supermarkets as their season is so fleeting. If you shop only in supermarkets you are missing out. There is rarely a need to buy apples or pumpkins from outside the UK.

Some fruits have to be imported but resist those that are heavily packaged and pre-prepared; they will have lost nutritional content during their handling. Pesticides create higher levels of acidity in fruits and vegetables so buy organic. If the extra cost puts you off, bear in mind that you will be spending far less on your usual shopping. Just not buying coffee for a week will help you meet the difference in cost.

We follow the seasons because each food has its growing cycle and a time when it is at its best, not just in terms of taste, but also its nutrition. We wait for the sun-warmed strawberries to appear in May. You can get winter vitamin C from rhubarb, nettles and wild garlic, or buy the tropical fruits as a winter treat. In autumn the alkaline root vegetables carrots, beetroots and celeriac are at their best. Foods in season are at their most economical too.

Use your freezer to make the most of seasonal fruit. A few forays to go blackberry, strawberry or raspberry picking is a good opportunity to stock up the freezer ready for juicing in the weeks ahead.

If you like to buy food in bulk check that you plan to use it all within a few days; it is easy to get bored with a whole bag of carrots. Fruit and vegetables can lose appeal and nutrients as they go past their best. However, the way supermarkets work it can be much cheaper to, say, buy a whole watermelon than a packaged slice.

SHOPPING LIST

	FRESH FRUIT, VEGETABLES, HERBS	FRIDGE, STORECUPBOARD
DAY 1	½ grapefruit, 1 lemon, 1 red apple, 3 red radishes, handful of baby spinach leaves, 4 carrots, ½ lime, 1 broccoli floret, 1 parsnip or sweet potato, 2 onions, 1 leek, 2 potatoes, 3 cloves garlic, 9 stalks celery, 1½ cucumbers, 2 cm ginger root, 2 bunches of parsley	1 teaspoon flaxseed, pumpkin or avocado oil, 12 almonds, skin on, 6 black peppercorns, 1 bay leaf, sea or rock salt, olive oil
DAY 2	1 pink grapefruit, 1 lemon, 1 lime, 1 orange, 50 g raspberries, 50 g blueberries, 1 beetroot and 3 beetroot leaves, 3 carrots, 2 onions, 2 stalks celery, 1 leek, 2 potatoes, 1 parsnip or sweet potato, bunch of spring onions, 150g fresh or frozen shelled peas, 1 spring mint, 2 cm piece of ginger root, parsley leaves	125 ml coconut water, fresh if possible, 1 teaspoon honey or 2 stevia leaves, 1 teaspoon walnut, almond or olive oil, 2 tablespoons chia seeds
DAY 3	1 small mango, 1 small green or pink apple, 1 green apple, ½ lime, 50 g blackcurrants or other berries, 3 handfuls of spinach leaves, 3 leaves kale, 3 leaves green cabbage, handful bean sprouts	250 ml milk or almond milk, 2 tablespoons double cream, 140 g rolled oats, about 4 cm cinnamon bark, fresh nutmeg
DAY 4	1 banana, 1 green apple, 8 fresh lychees, ½ green pepper, 1 Swiss chard leaf, 3 red cabbage leaves, 6 chicory leaves, 3 romaine lettuce leaves, 3 beetroot leaves, 6 sprigs of watercress, 1 cauliflower, 1 leek, 2 stalks celery, handful of coriander	250 ml aloe vera juice, 2 tablespoons flaxseeds, 2 tablespoons sunflower or pumpkin seeds, 12 almonds, skin on, 1 tablespoon sesame seeds, handful of dried wild mushrooms
DAY 5	1 pear, 1 grapefruit, 1 orange, 1 lemon, 1 small or ½ avocado, 1 lime, 2 red plums, 1 small sweet potato, 3 romaine lettuce leaves, ½ fennel bulb, 150 g fresh spinach, 1 celery stalk, 1 onion, 1 leek, handful of spinach leaves, 5 carrots, 3 sprigs of mint, 2 sprigs of lemon thyme, small bunch of parsley	250 ml elderflower tea, 1 tablespoon double cream, 1 teaspoon honey or 2 stevia leaves, 1 teaspoon spirulina, sea or rock salt
DAY 6	slice of watermelon (about ⅛th), 1 lime, 1 small avocado, 1 lemon, 5 cm slice of pineapple, 1 peach or nectarine, 1 orange, 1 large tomato, 1 celery stalk with leaves, 1 potato, 50 g cabbage, 3 beetroots, 1 cucumber, 2 fresh red or green chillies (about 2 cm long), 1 sprig of mint, 2 stems of coriander	coconut water (optional), 1 tablespoon crème fraîche, 1 teaspoon apple cider vinegar, sea or rock salt, 1 tablespoon olive oil
DAY 7	1 avocado, 1 lemon, 3 limes, handful of rocket leaves, handful spinach, 1 cucumber, 1 beetroot, 1 onion, 4 celery stalks, 1 carrot, small bunch of parsley, handful of coriander, 5 stems mint, 1 cm horseradish, 1 cm ginger	1 tablespoon butter (optional), 3 teaspoons flaxseeds, pumpkin or olive oil, 1 tablespoon curry paste, 2 tablespoons hemp seeds, 3 stevia leaves, 400 ml full-fat coconut milk, 400 ml coconut water, few almonds

CHOOSING YOUR EQUIPMENT

It is worth knowing that not all juicers are equal. New powerful juicers will make juicing easy for you. The best juicers can extract juice from leaves and give you the maximum possible nutrition from your ingredients. From a health point of view those are the big breakthroughs.

You may find that your old juicer, or one you have borrowed, struggles with beetroot, carrots and some leaves, but we'd rather you have a go and find out rather than put yourself off at the thought of buying something expensive. Some of the recipes in the book will work with a blending wand or a hand-press. Others will be hard work without a powerful juicer. Have a go.

Be careful with the last ingredient you juice. If you don't clean your machine every time you use it you can find some lingering liquid still left in the tube. The shortcut is to turn the motor on and wash out the machine with a glass of water until it runs clear before you start.

Centrifugal juicers

A centrifugal juicer (fig. 2 and 4) works by spinning the ingredients; it spits out the debris one way and the juice the other. They are not as good with leafy vegetables as the new powerful masticating juicers. The main disadvantage compared to a masticating juicer is that this method tends to let more oxygen in, so the nutrients degrade more quickly. If you use a centrifugal juicer it is best to drink your juice straight after juicing to get the most benefit. Choose a trusted long-standing brand as there quite a few duds out there.

Masticating juicers

A juicing machine is the best choice for juicing vegetables and hard fruits. A masticating model (fig. 1) 'chews' up your ingredients and some tests have shown that the nutritional content remains higher using this kind of juicer because they let less oxygen in than centrifugal models. New juicers are noticeably better than even just a few years ago because they produce more liquid per vegetable. If you are thinking of buying a new juicer it might help to know that you can use it for many cooking uses such as making purées, nut butters and ice creams. You can make a vegetable juice to add to soup, making your usual soup even more nutritious.

Vertical slow juicers are the most affordable and easily available. They are especially good for leafy greens and can even whizz up wheatgrass. Twin gear juices are slower than vertical and more expensive, but some say the

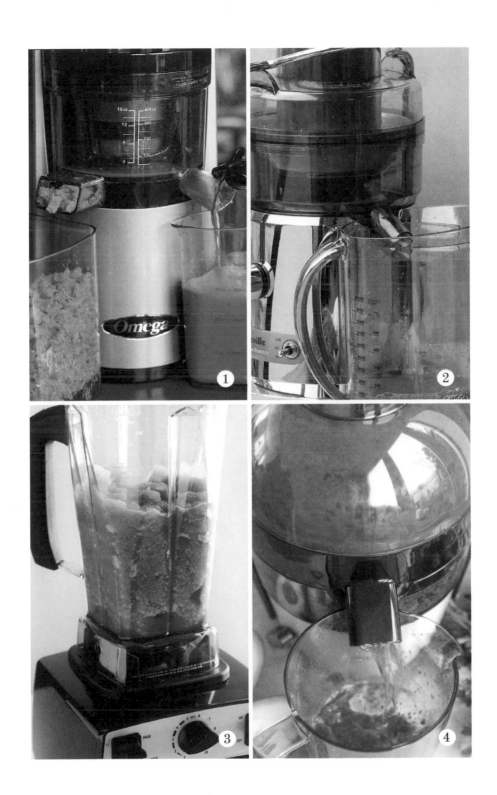

juice is better. Nutritionists often recommend them. Horizontal single-blade masticating juicers are like old-fashioned mincing machines, crushing the vegetables through a stainless steel mesh. They tend to be cheaper and are good for greens.

Blending wand

Hand wands are affordable and will be able to blend soups and fresh fruit smoothies pretty effectively. Your wand might also manage some greens in there too, as long as you are not asking it to juice a huge amount. It might struggle with frozen fruits. You will need a thin tall jug that it can fit inside easily along with your ingredients. Some are sold with a jug but it might not be big enough for some of the recipes in the book, such as the soups; find one that works for you.

Stand food processor

If you already own (or can borrow) a food processor or blender (fig. 3) you will be able to make the soups and some of the smoothies. If the recipe contains some liquid, such as apple juice, water or coconut milk, a food processor will work fine whizzing up soft fruit, a chopped green vegetable and maybe a ripe apple, but it won't help with the big valuable vegetables like carrots and beetroot. If you cook the vegetables first, as in the soup recipes, a food processor will cope with liquidising soups.

Wheatgrass juicer

Twin-gear, single drill or screw-type juicers are best for wheatgrass and other leafy greens because they operate at the lower speeds needed to deal with fibrous leaves. The disadvantage is they tend to take longer. You can buy hand-operated wheatgrass juicers if you like a daily shot.

Citrus juicer

Oranges, lemons, grapefruits and other citrus fruits are probably best allocated a machine of their own, so you can avoid having to peel. A old-fashioned glass hand-squeezer will do the job perfectly well, then simply pour the juice into your other ingredients.

Electric squeezers do the work well and are often affordable. Choose a model where you hold the fruit down on the rotating head so you get all the juice. You can juice pomegranates using an electric squeezer – but watch out for the mess. Making your own citrus juice is far better than using commercial juices where the vitamins will have died during pasteurisation.

FREQUENTLY ASKED QUESTIONS

Will I have enough calories for my busy day?
The chances are that you consume too many calories already, so a few days downsizing might be a recommendation. Following the cleanse for between one and seven days will help to retrain your stomach so that you don't require as much food, while still providing you with enough fibre and nutrients to keep your body and mind happy.

How can I make this fit into my work life?
Juices are always at their best soon after they are made, as the vitamins and minerals tend to oxidise with time. However, taking a flask or bottle to work is easy. Prepping the night before means that they won't be left in the fridge for too long, and is actually much quicker than cooking a meal or making sandwiches. Or you can invest in a juicer for the office.

How many times a year should I do *The Alkaline Cleanse*?
The plan is to get you juicing. Once you have got the habit you can work the recipes into your everyday life and get the benefits of better nutrition, better food and an easier time in the kitchen. If you are feeling sluggish, one or two days of cleansing every few months can help to keep you going.

Can I do *The Alkaline Cleanse* if I am pregnant or have health issues?
Juicing equals healthy food, so get the habit early and enjoy it. However, you should consult a doctor before embarking on any major dietary change if you are pregnant.

Can I do the Seven-Day Cleanse for more than seven days?
How many days you cleanse for is up to you, but we wouldn't advise you to continue for much longer – seven days should be enough to get your digestion back to its natural state.

What if I slip up or take a day off during the plan?
Don't worry – if you have to go out for a meal, or can't make one of the recipes, just remember to rebalance the next day. This isn't a strict plan, it's the first steps towards a way of life, so there are bound to be some hiccups along the way.

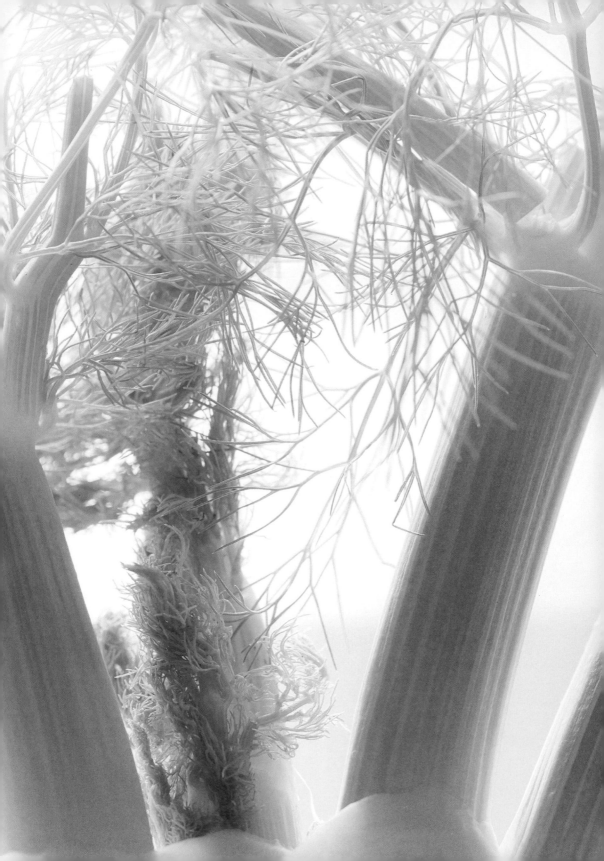

3
The Seven-Day Cleanse

Starting the Seven-Day Cleanse

Days One to Seven

STARTING THE SEVEN-DAY CLEANSE

OK there is no going back now. You have bought the book and have had a look on the internet to see if this cleanse is going to work. It works. You have worked out how to work the juicer. You are about to go out and buy lots of fruits and vegetables.

If you need a little push then think about this: you are going to feel a lot better and you are going to look a lot better. Your eyes are going to be clear and will sparkle. Your skin will look radiant and your digestive system is going to work like never before. You are going to enjoy some amazing new tastes and flavours and enjoy the variety of new recipes. Oh, and you will probably lose a little weight too.

How you might feel on the cleanse
The first few days of the cleanse may feel like uncharted territory while you get rid of your usual eating habits. On the first morning your reaction might be: what happened to my cup of coffee? And: why don't I have a croissant anyway? That is a very natural reaction and at this point you need to remind yourself about the reason you picked up this book.

The reason you just juiced the citrus fruits and celery is to cleanse your body of toxins and to give yourself a huge boost of vitamins and nutrients. Your body won't tell you about the benefits yet; that will take a few days to kick in, but stick with it. Our bodies don't change quickly; they take time to get used to a new routine. The message from the stomach and digestive system takes a while to get to the brain and back again, so be patient while your body gets used to what is going on.

There is no need to feel hungry on the cleanse. If you feel hungry or tired have a cup of Vegetable Tea (see page 57). Sip it slowly and remind yourself of the goodness you are giving your body.

Be patient with yourself while you get used to the new way of eating. You have to make space in your head to allow your body get rid of the toxins it has built up over the years.

Making the Seven-Day Cleanse work for you

Remember that the time spent making your juices, smoothies and soups, and the time you take to eat them, is important. This is your time to enjoy what you are creating and putting into your body, so don't rush. Enjoy it – make it an occasion. During a busy day at the office, 30 minutes to eat lunch will make the difference to both your digestive system and your mental wellbeing.

Thinking about the routine and rhythm of your day will help you achieve your cleanse goals. You can establish signposts that structure your day and help you notice how well you are doing. A few simple strategies can help you make the cleanse an easy and enjoyable part of your day:

*   Appreciate the beauty of your ingredients by giving them pride of place in the kitchen. Try out different combinations, or play with recipes you already know. Have fun with the nourishing fruits and vegetables you have bought.

*   Make your Vegetable Tea the night before. Make sure you have plenty so there is a cup ready for you if you get thirsty or hungry.

*   Set out, and if possible prepare, the ingredients for your breakfast while you make your Vegetable Tea so that they are ready for you in the morning.

*   While you prepare your breakfast, sip a glass of hot water with a few drops of fresh grapefruit or other citrus juice added. Take your time to drink it slowly.

*   Prepare your body and mind for each meal by setting a time to eat – and sticking to it.

*   Try not to eat last thing at night; your body needs time to digest food before you settle for sleep.

*   If you are working, you might be able to take your juicer to work. If not, make the juice or smoothie in the morning, keep it in the fridge at work, and give it a shake before you drink it. Take time to sip it slowly.

*   Always clean up after juicing so you don't return to a messy kitchen. Your equipment is easiest to clean just after use too.

DAY ONE

menu plan

Breakfast
Good Morning Juice

Lunch
Green Herbal Cleanser

Dinner
Vegetable Tea

Extra Shot
Almond and Broccoli Shot

You have taken the decision to reboot your body and begin your journey to good health and renewed vitality. Now that you understand the principles of an alkaline life, and have learnt about the delicious drinks and soups you will be making, you can start the plan. Check off all the items on your shopping list (see page 43) and get your juicer out ready, along with a big saucepan to make Vegetable Tea. Remember to sip your juices and soup and to savour each mouthful. Have the Almond and Broccoli Shot mid-morning or mid-afternoon to give you a protein-packed burst of energy. Sip water throughout the day too.

FOODS IN FOCUS

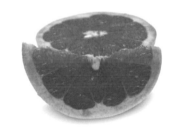

The first day focuses on preparing your body for the week ahead. The simple juice for breakfast contains detoxifying fruits, ginger and alkaline herbs to cleanse your gut. Grapefruits are full of vitamins and dietary fibre, which, along with the calming effects of ginger, will help to soothe your digestive system.

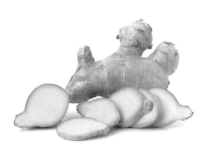

Herbs are the star in the lunch juice. Use whatever is in season; parsley is always a good choice and is a powerful antioxidant. A nutrient-rich Almond and Broccoli Shot will give you an energy boost. A gentle Vegetable Tea broth in the evening will allow an over-burdened stomach to rest. You will be set up, satisfied and ready for the rest of the week.

GOOD MORNING JUICE

For day one we need a cleansing juice to clear out the system. The red apple adds sweetness to counter the grapefruit and you also squeeze in a few salad vegetables for a nutrient-packed start to the day.

½ grapefruit
1 lemon
2 stalks celery
½ cucumber

3 red radishes
1 red apple
2 cm ginger root

Peel the grapefruit and lemon – leave a little pith and skin because it is richer in minerals and fibre than the fruit itself. Juice the grapefruit and lemon. Juice the celery. Peel the cucumber (especially if it has been waxed) and juice.

Juice the radishes; if the radish leaves are still fresh and green they can go in there too. Quarter the apple and juice. Peel the ginger root and drop it in to the juicer for a spicy kick. Mix well together, then pour into a glass to serve.

NOTE: You can add any leftover celery to your Vegetable Tea tonight.

MINDFUL MOTIVATION

*Eating requires a tranquil moment.
Take your time. Enjoy it. Don't gulp or
rush your food.*

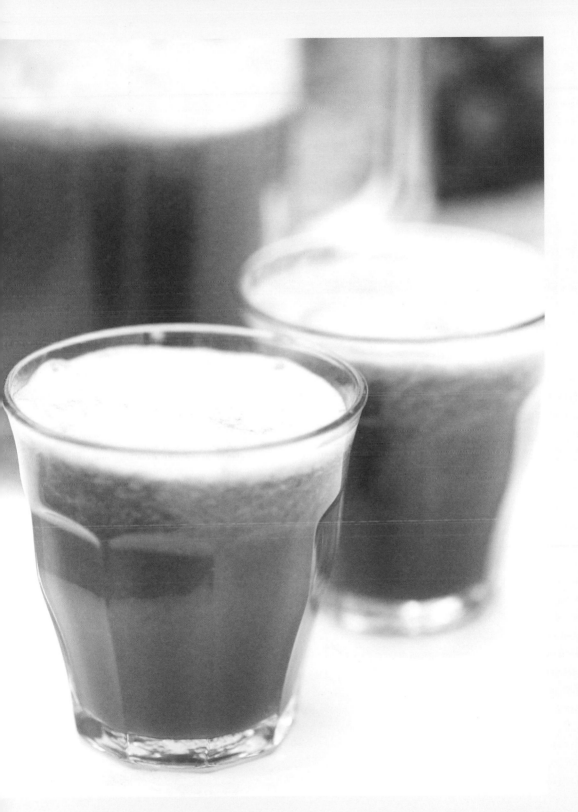

GREEN HERBAL CLEANSER

This is known as The Herbal Alchemist at the clinic. Fresh herbs have many attributes and we use them generously – both the stalks and leaves. We mix and change herbs through the seasons, starting with wild garlic and lovage in the summer. Use what you have to hand that is in season. Here we are using parsley but any of the gentler herbs like coriander are a good alternative or even, sparingly, a few thyme leaves or one or two sage leaves.

3 stalks celery, with leaves
handful of baby spinach leaves
small bunch of parsley
1 carrot

1 cucumber
½ lime
1 teaspoon flaxseed, pumpkin or
   avocado oil, to serve

Wash any dirt off the celery, spinach and parsley. Pat dry. Juice the celery. Top and tail the carrot and juice. Peel the cucumber and add to the juicer, followed by the spinach. Pick off the parsley leaves and add to the mix with the parsley stalks. Pour out the juice, mix well, and add a good squeeze of the lime. Pour into a glass to serve with the oil poured over.

ALMOND AND BROCCOLI SHOT

Try drinking this shot for a mid-morning or mid-afternoon snack. The almonds are packed full of healthy fats and energy-giving protein. Alter the amount of water to your own taste.

12 almonds, skin on
75 ml water

1 broccoli floret

Mix the almonds and the water first to break the nuts down.
Add the broccoli. Blend well.

☾ VEGETABLE TEA

This broth will do you the power of good and keep you full of energy. Make as much as you like because you can drink it throughout the day instead of caffeinated teas and coffees. Once you get the hang of making this tea vary the spices and herbs that you add to change the flavour; you can also try adding any leftover vegetables from other recipes. This base recipe will be the foundation of your evening meal soup tomorrow.

2 litres water
3 carrots
1 parsnip or sweet potato
4 stalks celery
2 onions
1 leek
2 potatoes

3 cloves garlic
6 black peppercorns
1 bay leaf
small bunch of parsley
sea or rock salt, to taste
olive oil, to serve

Put the water on to boil while you prepare the vegetables.

Trim and peel the carrots and parsnip or sweet potato and cut into large pieces. Roughly chop the celery. Peel and quarter the onions. Remove the root end of the leek and discard, and roughly chop the leek. Quarter the potatoes (there is no need to peel unless they are old and dirty).

When the water reaches boiling, add all the vegetables and the garlic, peppercorns and bay leaf. Cut the leaves off the parsley and put to one side. Roughly chop the parsley stalks and add to the vegetables. Cover and reduce the heat until the liquid is simmering, and cook for 30 minutes.

Strain the vegetables, keeping only the liquid. Warm the tea through when you want to drink it, and season to taste with sea or rock salt. Serve with a few parsley leaves placed on top and a little olive oil poured over, if you like.

TIP: Parsley is surprisingly strong and peppery when juiced. You can juice the leaves and drizzle a swirl on top for an extra healthy chlorophyl kick.

DAY TWO

menu plan

Breakfast
Grapefruit, Lemon and Lime Juice

Lunch
Vitality Juice

Dinner
Alkaline Minestrone Soup

Extra Shot
Coconut, Chia and Berry Blast

Congratulations! You've made it through your first day. Notice how your body feels. Perhaps you're already feeling lighter, less bloated? You might be a little more hungry than usual, too, especially when you wake up. It might come as a surprise because you've never been a breakfast person. These are good signs. Your body is shifting gears. It's time to nourish yourself again.

FOODS IN FOCUS

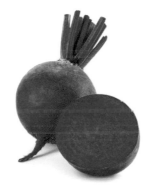

Day two is about boosting your body's ability to fight inflammation and oxidation through foods high in antioxidant-rich vitamin C, as well as cleansing the blood and liver with potent nutrients found in beets. The naturally occuring electrolyte, potassium, in the coconut-water-based shot should help keep you hydrated and provide a good dose of minerals as well as B-vitamins to keep your energy levels up.

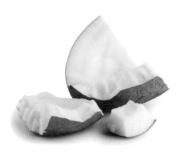

If you are finding it hard to go without caffeine, use green tea instead of coconut water in the Coconut, Chia and Berry Blast. Green tea is high in antioxidants but has a slight diuretic effect because it contains caffeine, so you might want to drink an extra cup of water or Vegetable Tea today. Your evening meal is jam-packed with vegetables, which your body will love.

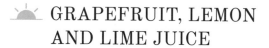

GRAPEFRUIT, LEMON AND LIME JUICE

Pink grapefruit is sweeter than yellow grapefruit but is just as refreshing and is packed with vitamin C. Sweeten if you like with a little honey or a few stevia leaves. This is a good exercise in diluting strong drinks and making them last longer; many commercial juices are sold too thick for our digestive systems.

1 pink grapefruit
1 lemon
1 lime

1 teaspoon honey or 2 stevia
    leaves, optional
125 ml water
1 spring mint

You can make this by hand using a citrus press; cut the fruits in half and hand-squeeze. If using a juicer, peel the grapefruit, lemon and lime and discard any pips. Divide into segments and place in the juicer. Add the honey or stevia leaves, if using, to your juice, and mix well. Pour into a glass and top with the water. Pick the mint leaves off the sprig and place in a bowl or mortar and crush with a pestle, muddler or wooden spoon to let the oils run. Add to the juice as a garnish.

NOTE: Naturally sweet, stevia leaves are a great alternative to sugar. Add the leaves to juices and smoothies if you need to.

MINDFUL MOTIVATION

Balance is everything in life. If we are too acidic we need to become more alkaline. Exercise, rest and the right foods at the right times can realign us to our natural rhythms.

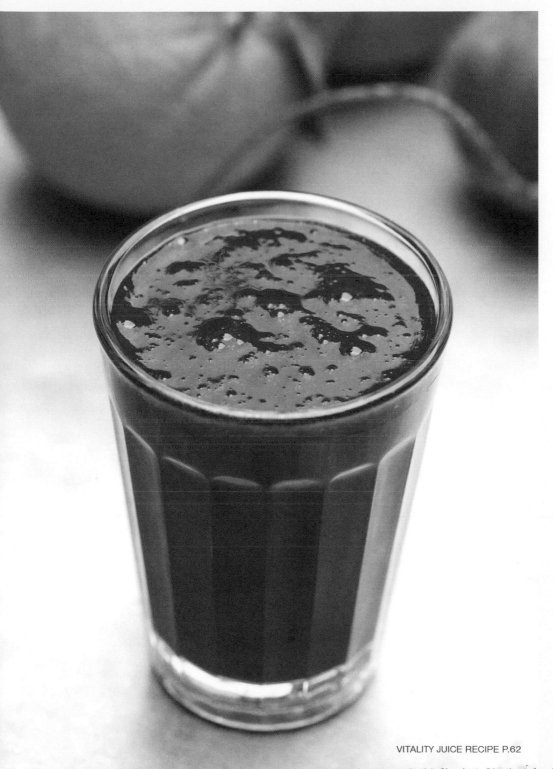

VITALITY JUICE RECIPE P.62

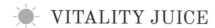 # VITALITY JUICE

Beetroot has blood-cleansing and detoxifying benefits – if they are fresh, the leaves especially so. The vitamin C in the orange provides antioxidants and ginger will give your digestive system a boost too. You could swap ginger for horseradish in autumn. If you have walnut oil use a little here; it especially loves beetroot.

1 orange
1 beetroot and 3 beetroot leaves
2 cm piece of ginger root

1 teaspoon walnut, almond or
   olive oil, to serve

Peel and divide the orange into segments. Peel and roughly chop the beetroot into crescents. Place in the juicer and juice. Peel the ginger root and add to the juicer. Mix well and pour into a glass. Pour over the oil to serve.

COCONUT, CHIA AND BERRY BLAST

Make the most of the precious water from a young coconut with this quick drink. If you are buying cartons of coconut water or milk read the cartons carefully; try not to choose the products with additives. Blending chia seeds makes them easier to digest. Berries add a burst of colour and summery flavour – you can vary this recipe by using papaya, cantaloupe melon or mango instead. You could also swap or mix the water with cold green tea.

125 ml coconut water,
fresh if possible
2 tablespoons chia seeds

50 g raspberries
50 g blueberries
125 ml water

Place everything into a blender. Whizz for a minute until smooth.
Check the taste and add more coconut water or plain water if
you like. Pour into a glass to serve.

☾ ALKALINE MINESTRONE SOUP

As you will be eating the vegetables in this soup, you need to cut the vegetables more neatly than during your preparation of the Vegetable Tea from day one. The soup does not have a long cooking time so the nutrients stay in the vegetables and they retain their texture.

1 litre Vegetable Tea (see day
   one, page 57)
3 carrots
2 onions
2 stalks celery
1 leek

2 potatoes
1 parsnip or sweet potato
bunch of spring onions
150 g fresh or frozen
   shelled peas
parsley leaves, to serve

Bring the Vegetable Tea to a simmer while you prepare the vegetables.

Trim and peel the carrots and dice. Peel the onions and cut into slices. Slice the celery. Cut off the root end of the leek and discard, and slice the leek into rings. Peel the potatoes and the parsnip or sweet potato, and dice.

Add the carrots, onions, celery, leek, potatoes and parsnip or sweet potato to the hot tea and simmer for 15 minutes until the vegetables have softened.

Cut off the root ends of the spring onions and discard. Slice the spring onions thinly and add to the soup along with the peas. Cook for a further five minutes. Ladle the soup into a bowl, and add a few parsley leaves to serve.

DAY THREE

menu plan

Breakfast
Porridge with Mango and Cinnamon

Lunch
Popeye's Juice

Dinner
Green Minestrone Soup

Extra Shot
Apple and Blackcurrant Crush

Day three is probably the hardest of the week. You might feel lethargic and tired especially if you've been relying on caffeine to get through your days – you might even have a slight headache. To help lift your mood you'll enjoy a big breakfast of Porridge with Mango and Cinnamon and a green Popeye's Juice for lunch. To clear your mind, go for a walk outside and breathe deeply to feed your brain and organs some extra oxygen.

FOODS IN FOCUS

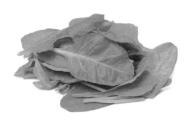

Remember, the foods you've been eating are designed to rid your body of toxins. As this happens feeling a little tired or headachey is normal. The slow-burn oats in the breakfast Porridge with Mango and Cinnamon will keep your hunger at bay, give you some needed comfort and help regulate your blood sugar levels throughout the morning. Cinnamon will aid digestion and lift the mood.

For lunch you will enjoy Popeye's Juice with kale and spinach. Spinach is rich in nutrients. You have it again for dinner and the addition of crème fraîche will make it taste luxurious and satisfying.

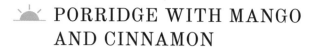 # PORRIDGE WITH MANGO AND CINNAMON

After a couple of days of juices and soups it is comforting to have an old-fashioned and reassuring porridge. You can use amaranth and quinoa instead of oats if you prefer. The carotenes in mango are a calming influence on the stomach, as well as being very good for skin.

140 g rolled oats
250 ml milk or almond milk

1 small mango
about 4 cm cinnamon bark

Put the oats in a non-stick pan and heat to toast lightly for a minute. Add the milk and stir. Increase the heat and cook for about three minutes or until the porridge starts to bubble and pop, then set aside.

Peel the mango and whizz in a blender until smooth. Using a pestle and mortar break up the cinnamon into a fine dust. Pour the porridge into a bowl (add more milk if you like) and top with the mango and cinnamon.

MINDFUL MOTIVATION

*Take time to appreciate what you are eating.
A mango takes many months to grow.
Show it respect. Enjoy the preparation
as much as the consumption.*

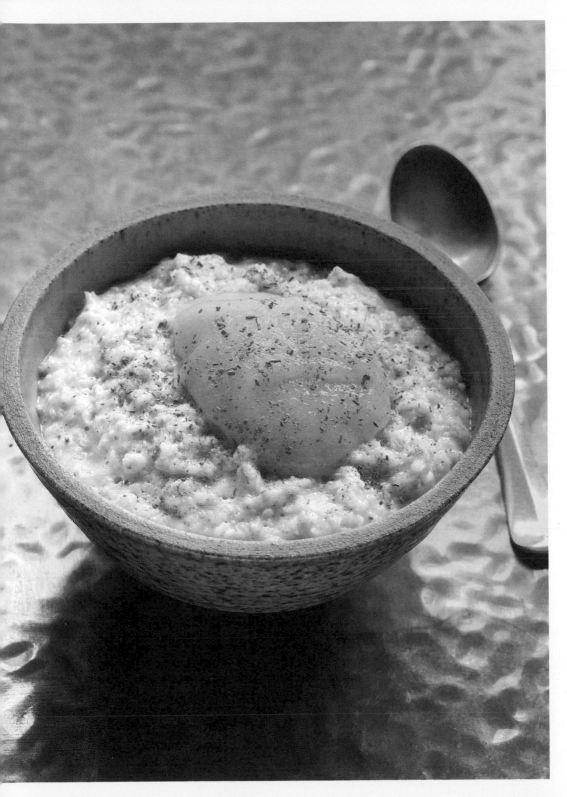

POPEYE'S JUICE

Cruciferous vegetables such as kale and cabbage are a great source of plant-based vitamins, minerals and cancer-fighting phytonutrients. They also have cholesterol-lowering properties, which are enhanced by light steaming when consumed whole.

½ lime
3 leaves kale
1 green apple

handful bean sprouts
handful baby spinach
3 green cabbage leaves
ice cubes, optional, to serve

Peel the lime and remove the stalks from the kale. Chop the apple into chunks and remove the core. Juice all the ingredients and serve over ice, if using.

APPLE AND BLACKCURRANT CRUSH

Apple and blackcurrant is one of the most popular drink combinations, but commercial products are often made with reconstituted juices – which is why they have vitamins added. Blackcurrants are ideal when in season but other berries such as strawberry, raspberry and gooseberry also make stunning combinations with apple.

1 small green or pink apple
50 g blackcurrants or other berries

125 ml water

Cut the apple in half and discard the core and pips. Place all the ingredients in a blender and whizz for one minute until smooth.

☾ GREEN MINESTRONE SOUP

The art of clever soup making is changing one recipe into another. This is a very easy trick that transforms yesterday's busy minestrone into a completely different smooth green emulsion with the extra benefits of all the magnesium in the spinach. It is also very quick – just the time to warm the pan and wilt the greens – but no less delicious or healthy for being convenient. Serve with a small chunk of rye or spelt bread

½ litre of Alkaline Minestrone
  Soup (see page 63)
2 handfuls of spinach leaves

2 tablespoons crème fraîche
fresh nutmeg, to serve

Heat the Alkaline Minestrone Soup to warm through. As it starts to simmer add the spinach leaves and stir in until the spinach is submerged in the soup. When the spinach starts to wilt, after about two minutes, remove the pan from the heat.

Transfer the soup to a blender or liquidiser and whizz until smooth. Add the crème fraîche and stir through. Ladle into a bowl and grate over a little nutmeg to taste.

DAY FOUR

menu plan

Breakfast
Nut and Seed Milk

Lunch
Gerson's Greens

Dinner
Cauliflower and Wild Mushroom Consommé

Extra Shot
Lychee and Aloe Vera Cooler

You're over the hump! How are you feeling? Today is going to be a super-healthy day full of seeds and a variety of vegetables, including some cancer-fighting greens. Why not enjoy some gentle stretches first thing in the morning to get your blood flowing. You should feel more energised right away. In the afternoon go for a brisk walk or do a short yoga session and follow it with a rehydrating Lychee and Aloe Vera Cooler.

FOODS IN FOCUS

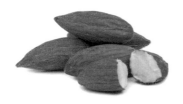

It's time to give your digestive system another boost. Today our focus turns to a new group of foods: nuts and seeds. They are rich in good fats and amino-acids. They also contain plenty of fibre, so you will make Nut and Seed Milk which is easy to digest.

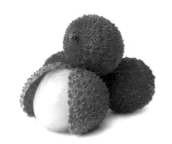

The famous Gerson's Greens drink at lunch contains six types of leaves, giving you an amazing variety of nutrients. The Lychee and Aloe Vera Cooler is rich in potassium and vitamin C. Tonight's delicious Cauliflower and Wild Mushroom Consommé will provide essential nutrients and add greatly to the day's hydration.

NUT AND SEED MILK

We start with a seed-packed cocktail of amino acids; the technique is the same as making almond milk but the cast of characters is bigger. You can vary the seeds you use and work out the ones you like best, using this recipe long after your Seven-Day Cleanse. We serve this with sliced banana on top which is great for breakfast, but you could try it with other fruits too.

350 ml water
2 tablespoons flaxseeds
2 tablespoons sunflower or
   pumpkin seeds

1 tablespoon sesame seeds
12 almonds, skin on
1 banana, to serve

Warm the water and then pour it over the seeds and nuts to cover. Leave for at least 10 minutes to plump up; overnight won't do them any harm. Pour everything into a blender and whizz for one minute. Serve in a bowl with the banana sliced over the top.

MINDFUL MOTIVATION

Eat small mouthfuls or take small sips at a time.
To be strict use a teaspoon to eat this nut milk.
Slow and steady gathers the nutrition.

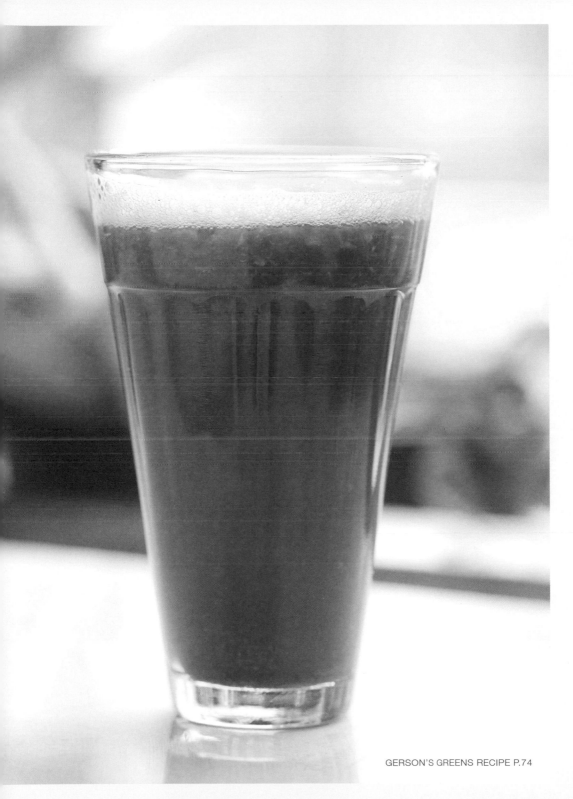

GERSON'S GREENS RECIPE P.74

GERSON'S GREENS

Max Gerson was an early pioneer of juicing to combat cancer and other chronic conditions. This is his classic recipe which is served every day at the San Diego Clinic in California. Green, tart apples are ideal and you do not peel the skin, keeping all the fibre in the juice. Ideally, use very fresh leaves; buy and use on the same day if possible.

½ green pepper
1 Swiss chard leaf
1 green apple
3 red cabbage leaves

6 chicory leaves
3 romaine lettuce leaves
3 beetroot leaves
6 sprigs of watercress

Cut the pepper in half and discard any seeds or pith and chop roughly. Remove the stalk from the chard leaf. Cut the apple in half and discard the core and pips. Cut it into rough chunks. Tear any large leaves in half and place all the ingredients in a juicer to juice. Mix well and pour into a glass to serve.

LYCHEE AND ALOE VERA COOLER

Lychees are a good source of potassium, antioxidants and vitamin C and are very good for your skin. Aloe vera is a rich source of essential amino acids and has both anti-inflammatory and immune-boosting properties. Aloe vera is tricky to juice so feel free to use the juice sold in cartons.

8 fresh lychees
250 ml aloe vera juice

cold water

Peel the lychees and discard the stones. Place in a blender with the aloe vera juice and whizz for one minute until smooth. Taste to check the strength and dilute with water if too strong. Pour into a glass to serve.

☾ CAULIFLOWER AND WILD MUSHROOM CONSOMMÉ

The soaking and cooking water is key here so don't fuss over chopping the vegetables beautifully as you won't be serving them in this consommé. Use a little of the cooked cauliflower as a garnish and use any leftover vegetables to make more Vegetable Tea or purée the cauliflower to serve as a side dish.

handful of dried wild mushrooms
1 cauliflower
1 leek
2 stalks celery

handful of coriander
250 ml Vegetable Tea (see page 57)

If any mushrooms are larger than a soup spoon, snip them in half using scissors. Place the mushrooms in a bowl and pour over enough boiling water to cover. Leave to soak for about 15 minutes until the mushrooms are reconstituted.

Place the cauliflower whole into a large saucepan and pour over water to cover. Remove the root end of the leek and discard. Dice the leek and celery and add to the pan. Cut the leaves off the coriander and chop the stalks finely. Add the coriander stalks to the pan. Cover, bring to the boil, and simmer for 20 minutes until the cauliflower is soft. Drain, keeping all the liquid.

Transfer the mushrooms and their soaking liquid to a clean pan and add the Vegetable Tea. Add the cauliflower liquid, mix well, and heat to warm through. Ladle the soup into a bowl and add some of the cooked cauliflower. Serve with a few coriander leaves over the top.

DAY FIVE

menu plan

Breakfast
Wake-up Surprise

Lunch
Spirulina and Spinach Smoothie

Dinner
Potassium Broth

Extra Shot
Elderflower, Lime and Plum Cooler

By now you should be able to start seeing the effects of the cleanse. It's a good time to use a gentle exfoliator made with a little almond or olive oil and sea salt flakes to remove dead skin cells from your face and body and reveal that healthy glow your skin should now have. It's a good day for some meditation or self-reflection too; perhaps go for a walk and praise yourself for looking after your body.

FOODS IN FOCUS

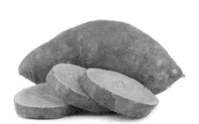

Today's menu is all about making your digestive system even more efficient so that all of the nutrients you eat can be more easily absorbed. Juiced sweet potato in the breakfast Wake-up Surprise will help to develop healthy gut flora (essential to proper digestion). The plums in the Elderflower, Lime and Plum Cooler will help keep your digestive cycle on time and in check.

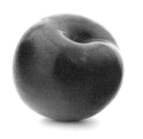

Spirulina and Spinach Smoothie for lunch is a powerful way to boost your immune system and contains useful protein. The evening's soup, rich in potassium, will help you feel grounded.

WAKE-UP SURPRISE

Sweet potatoes are very alkaline and make a satisfying, if a little unusual, start to the day. Other potatoes can cause gas if juiced raw but sweet potatoes are another story. The pear and carrot add a lovely sweetness as well as fibre and vitamins. The grapefruit adds a refreshing citrus hit for your morning juice.

1 small sweet potato	3 romaine lettuce leaves
1 pear	½ fennel bulb
1 carrot	1 grapefruit

Peel and chop the sweet potato, pear and carrot. Place in a juicer and juice. Add the romaine lettuce leaves, and juice. Slice the fennel into manageable pieces and juice. Peel the grapefruit, divide into segments and juice. Mix well, then pour into a glass to serve.

MINDFUL MOTIVATION

*The alkaline elements in the juices will help
to restore the natural flora in your gut.*

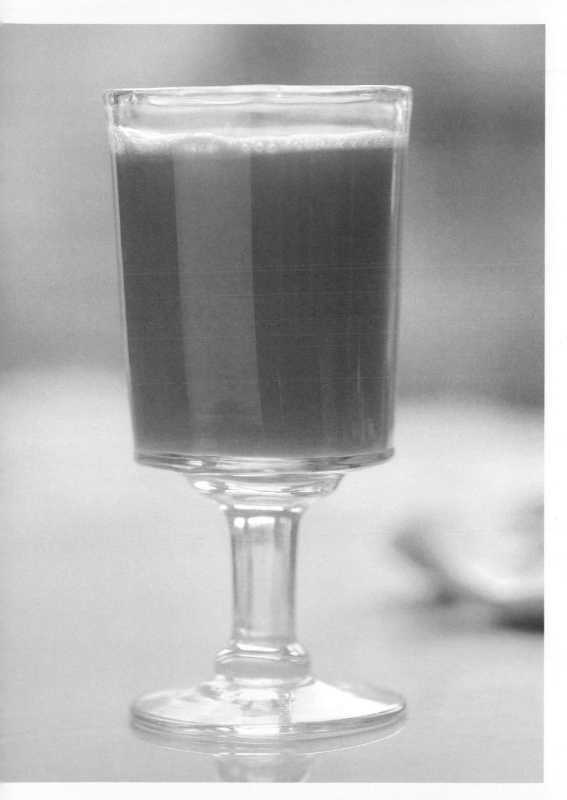

SPIRULINA AND SPINACH SMOOTHIE

Spirulina is a type of vibrant green sea algae that can help to boost your immune system; it was possibly the first living organism to photosynthesise light from the sun and was critical in starting life on earth. Along with creamy avocado and fresh spinach, this makes a healthful green lunch.

1 orange
1 lemon
1 small or ½ avocado
3 sprigs of mint
150 g fresh spinach

1 teaspoon honey or
   2 stevia leaves
1 teaspoon spirulina
cold water or ice cubes, optional

Peel the orange and lemon, cut the flesh into chunks, and discard any pips. Peel and stone the avocado. Pick the leaves off the mint. Place all the ingredients except the water or ice cubes in a blender and whizz for one minute until smooth. Add water or ice to dilute if too sludgey and pour into a glass to serve.

ELDERFLOWER, LIME AND PLUM COOLER

The sweet and sour combination of lime and plum juices goes really well with the grounding aroma of elderflower and lemon thyme. Fibre in the plum is good for maintaining a regular digestive cycle.

1 lime
2 red plums

2 sprigs of lemon thyme
250 ml elderflower tea

Peel the lime, cut into chunks and discard any pips. Halve and stone the plums. Pick off the lemon thyme leaves and discard the woody stems. Place everything in a blender with the tea and whizz for one minute. Pour into a glass to serve.

☾ POTASSIUM BROTH

This recipe is based on a raw broth devised by juice pioneer Norman Walker. He considered carrots, parsley, spinach and celery to be outstanding ingredients. We cook the vegetables in this recipe to give you a hot, satisfying final meal of the day.

1 litre water
1 celery stalk
4 carrots
1 onion
1 leek

small bunch of parsley
handful of spinach leaves
sea or rock salt
1 tablespoon crème fraîche,
    to serve

Bring the water to a boil while you prepare the vegetables. Slice the celery into small crescents. Trim and peel the carrots and dice. Peel and slice the onion. Remove the root end of the leek and discard, and slice the leek into rings. Add the celery, carrots, onion and leek to the boiling water.

Cut the leaves off the parsley and put to one side. Chop the stalks and add to the broth. Simmer for 50 minutes. Remove from the heat then add the parsley leaves and spinach.

Transfer everything to a blender or liquidiser and whizz until smooth. Add a little salt to taste. Ladle into a bowl and add the crème fraîche to serve.

DAY SIX

menu plan

Breakfast
Watermelon, Cucumber and Mint Juice

Lunch
Salsa Smoothie

Dinner
Very Very Quick Borscht

Extra Shot
Pineapple Piña Colada

Today is all about a variety of colours. The more colourful the fruit and vegetable mix in your diet is, the more potent the sum of its nutritional benefits. It's a good day for some more strenuous exercise such as Pilates, hot yoga or light weights. A grounding and detoxifying beetroot soup for dinner should help you feel satiated.

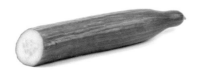

FOODS IN FOCUS

Today you will enjoy lycopene-rich red tomatoes; chlorophyll-rich cucumber, celery, mint and cabbage; and betacyanin-rich purple beets.

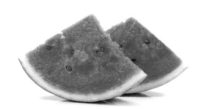

The watermelon breakfast juice is hydrating and zesty and will make a delicious start to the day. If you choose to do some strenuous exercise, have your Pineapple Piña Colada shot an hour before you start as it is high in vitamin C, manganese and vitamin B1 which are co-factors in the body's own energy production. Pineapple is also a good digestive aid.

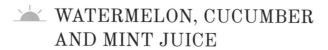 WATERMELON, CUCUMBER
AND MINT JUICE

This is delicious on a hot summer morning. The soft, water-packed watermelon and cucumber are very easy to blend and make a refreshing drink that is also packed with fibre. Make sure you include the watermelon seeds for their texture.

slice of watermelon (about ⅛)   1 lime
½ cucumber   1 sprig of mint

Cut the watermelon thinly. Peel the cucumber. Peel the lime and hand-squeeze the juice. Pick off about 15 mint leaves and put everything in a blender. Whizz until smooth.

TIP: If you keep the ingredients in the fridge overnight they will be cool when you want to use them so there is no need to add ice.

MINDFUL MOTIVATION

Fill your lungs with fresh air every day. They will thank you for it. Breathe deeply and exhale all those acid toxins.

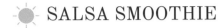 # SALSA SMOOTHIE

Summer in a glass. The riper the fruits the more alkaline they are, so take time to choose ingredients at their peak.

1 large tomato	1 fresh red or green chilli (about
½ cucumber	2 cm long)
1 celery stalk, with leaves	1 teaspoon apple cider vinegar
2 stems of coriander	sea or rock salt
1 small avocado	200 ml water
1 lemon	1 tablespoon olive oil, to serve

Roughly chop the tomato. Peel the cucumber and cut into large chunks. Chop the celery stalks and all the coriander, stalks included. Peel and stone the avocado. Peel the lemon, cut into chunks, and discard any pips. Put in a blender and whizz until smooth. Trim the chilli crossways, discard the seeds and membrane and chop finely. Add as much chilli as you like and whizz to combine. Add the apple cider vinegar, a little salt and the water. Mix well and pour into a glass. Pour over the olive oil to serve

PINEAPPLE PIÑA COLADA

In the Caribbean pineapple juice is always served diluted with ice and water to make it a longer drink. Chilli adds a little fire but is also alkaline; you only need to add a little chilli to counter the sweet pineapple.

5 cm slice of pineapple	70 ml water or coconut water
1 peach or nectarine	1 fresh red or green chilli
	(about 2 cm long)

Peel the slice of pineapple and cut out the hard central core. Cut the pineapple into cubes. Quarter the peach or nectarine and disard the stone. Place everything in a blender except the chilli and whizz until smooth. Trim the chilli crossways, discard the seeds and membrane and chop finely. Add as much chilli as you like and whizz to combine. Pour into a glass to serve.

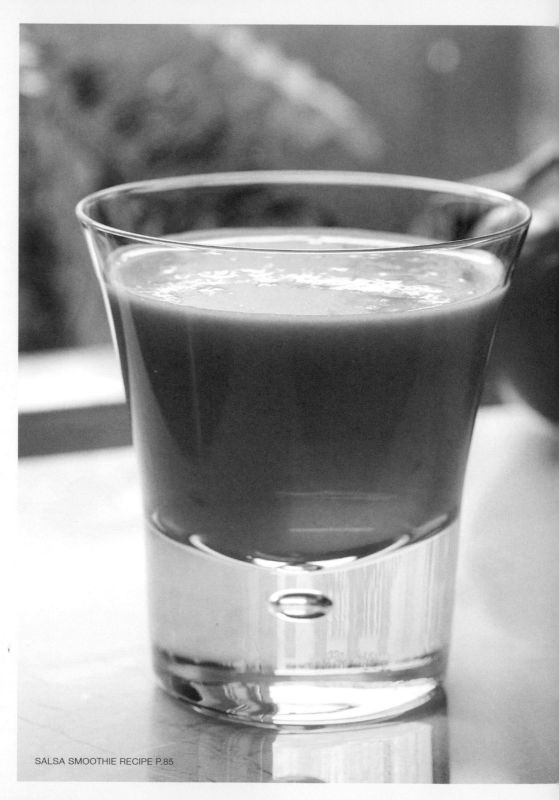

SALSA SMOOTHIE RECIPE P.85

☾ VERY VERY QUICK BORSCHT

This can be messy as you need to juice the beetroot first, but the results are worth it as this method keeps the magical deep ruby hues. It also saves about an hour of cooking time. You can blend if you like for a smooth borscht but if time is against you, there is no need.

1 potato	1 orange
50 g cabbage	1 tablespoon crème fraîche,
3 beetroots	to serve

Bring a saucepan of water to the boil. Cut the potato into quarters (there is no need to peel) and add to the pan. Simmer for about 10 minutes. Chop the cabbage and add, cooking for a further five minutes. Drain.

Peel the beetroots and grate one beetroot into a clean saucepan. Place the other two beetroots in a juicer and juice. Peel the orange, cut into chunks, and discard the pips. Add the orange to the juicer.

Pour the juice into the pan and bring to a simmer. Add the potatoes and cabbage, mix well, and cook for about five minutes. Blend if you have time. Ladle into a bowl with the crème fraîche spooned on top.

DAY SEVEN

menu plan

Breakfast
The Original FX Mayr Green Smoothie

Lunch
Rocket and Lime Herbal

Dinner
Carrot and Coconut Soup

Extra Shot
Beetroot and Horseradish Shot

You made it to the last day! How are you feeling? Your skin should be glowing and the whites of your eyes should have a bright sparkle. You might be surprised about this, but now that your body and digestive system have had time to heal and recalibrate, you might no longer be craving those sugary or processed treats. Feel free to do a final almond or olive oil and sea salt flakes body exfoliation to get rid of those toxins and reveal your fresh skin. When you have finished the week, think of which were your favourite recipes and try to include them as part of your usual diet. Perhaps continue to do at least one day of the plan every week.

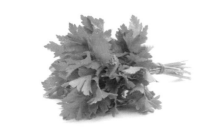

FOODS IN FOCUS

Today your digestive system will get its final tune up of the Seven-Day Cleanse with a classic green smoothie from the FX Mayr clinic and a potent Rocket and Lime Herbal lunch.

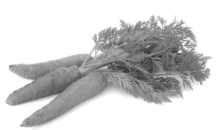

To celebrate your successful completion of the week we have prepared a wonderful carotenoid-rich Carrot and Coconut Soup for dinner tonight. Its creamy texture and slight sweetness from the carrot and coconut cream will make this a treat of a meal.

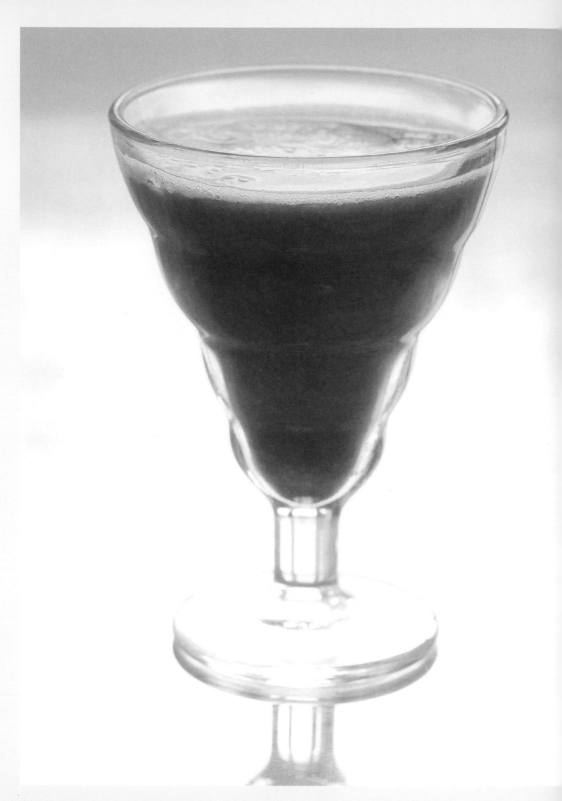

THE ORIGINAL FX MAYR GREEN SMOOTHIE

This is the famous green smoothie served at the Mayr Clinic in Austria. It contains plenty of great alkaline ingredients such as parsley and spinach as well as a rich cocktail of nutrients from the seeds and oil. You might find this sweet enough without the stevia leaves – you can taste before adding if you like.

½ cucumber
1 handful spinach
5 stems mint
5 stems parsley
1 cm ginger root
1 avocado

400 ml coconut water
1 lime
2 tablespoons flaxseed, pumpkin
   or olive oil
2 tablespoons hemp seeds
3 stevia leaves, optional

Peel the cucumber and add to a juicer with the spinach. Pick the leaves off the mint and parsley and add. Peel the ginger root and add. Transfer to a blender. Peel and stone the avocado, scoop out the flesh and add to the blender with the coconut water. Squeeze the lime and add the juice. Add the oil, hemp seeds and stevia, if using. Whizz together until smooth then pour into a glass to serve.

 # ROCKET AND LIME HERBAL

This is a real green tonic – if you have any fresh leaves from yesterday's beetroots add them too. Radish leaves are also good additions.

4 celery stalks
handful of rocket leaves
handful of fresh parsley

½ cucumber
1 lime
1 teaspoon flaxseed or olive oil

Place the celery stalks in a juicer and juice, followed by the rocket and parsley; use the leaves and stalks. Peel the cucumber and juice. Peel the lime, cut into chunks and discard any pips. Add to the juicer. Mix well and pour into a glass. Serve with the flaxseed or olive oil on top.

☾ CARROT AND COCONUT SOUP

This delicious soup only takes about fifteen minutes to cook so is a very useful recipe to have up your sleeve. The creamy coconut milk makes it a satisfying supper for the end of your cleanse. Well done – almost there!

1 onion
1 tablespoon butter, optional
1 tablespoon curry paste
200 g carrots
400 ml full-fat coconut milk

about 100 ml water
1 lime
few almonds, to garnish
handful of coriander, to garnish

Peel and dice the onion. Heat the butter, or if your coconut milk has a solid cream top, you can use that, and cook the onion for a few minutes until softened. Stir in the curry paste. Trim, peel and chop the carrots and add to the onions. Stir well. Add the coconut milk and enough water to cover. Simmer for 10 minutes. Transfer everything to a blender and blend until smooth.

Season the soup with a generous squeeze of lime juice. Toast the almonds lightly in a pan, then chop roughly. Chop the coriander. Serve the soup with the toasted almonds and chopped coriander scattered over.

BEETROOT AND HORSERADISH SHOT

A kick of heat from the horseradish will take your mind off any thoughts of hunger, and give you an alkaline boost.

1 beetroot
1 lemon

1 cm horseradish

Peel the beetroot and cut into crescents. Peel the lemon, cut into chunks and discard any pips. Put the beetroot and lemon in the juicer and juice. Grate the horseradish into the juice and mix well. Pour into a shot glass to serve.

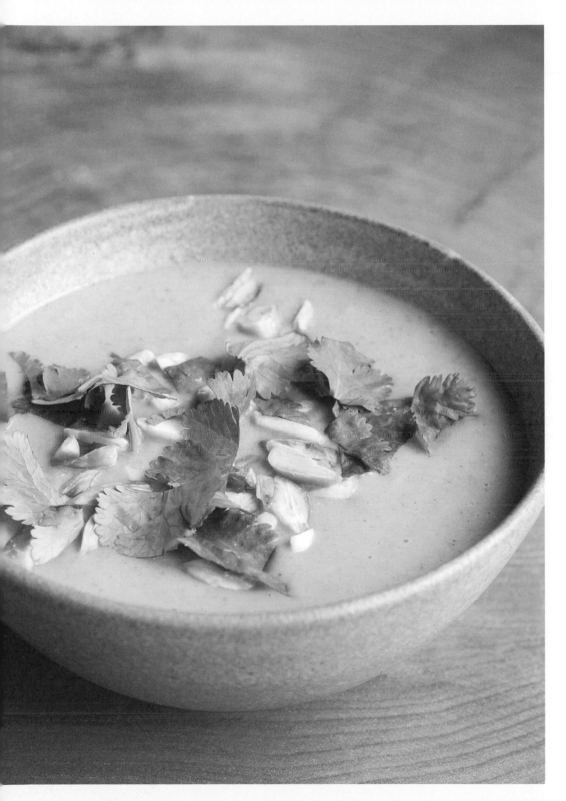

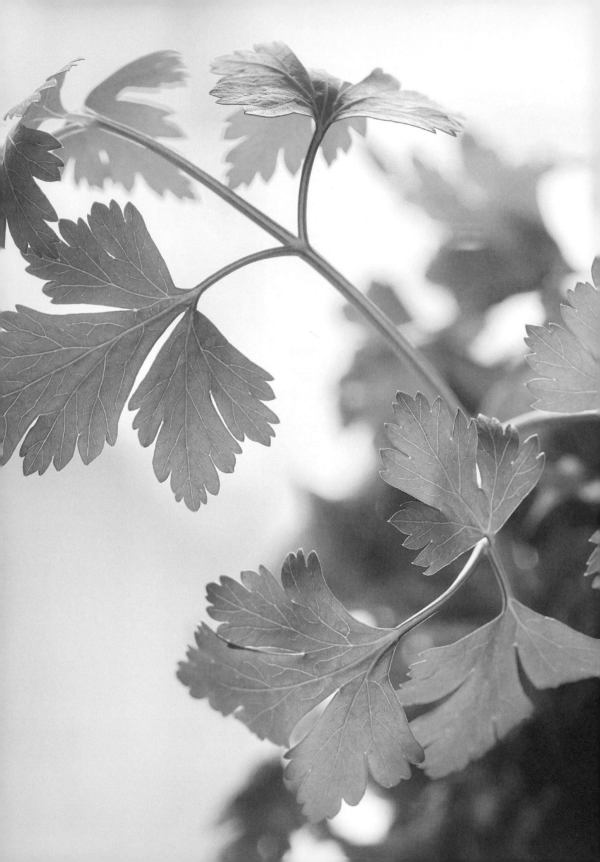

4
Cleansing for Life

Juices and Smoothies for Every Day

Fruit Juices and Smoothies

Green Juices and Smoothies

Vegetable Juices and Smoothies

Nutri-Boost Recipes

Teas and Tisanes

JUICES AND SMOOTHIES FOR EVERY DAY

Smoothies, juices and vegetable and herbal teas are a pleasure to drink and are an easy way to get fruits, vegetables, nuts and seeds and all their nutrients into your diet. Things that, let's be honest, most of us don't eat enough of in today's world of over-processed, pre-packaged food.

Quick, easy and good for you
All the recipes in the book are relatively inexpensive to make, but pack plenty of health benefits. Because they are made using a variety of raw whole foods, they can help alkalise the body, improve digestion, boost immunity and increase energy.

Most of the recipes take just a few minutes to make, can be transported easily and can be stored in the fridge for up to 12 hours, which means they can be taken to work. You can incorporate any of the recipes as meal replacements – whether for breakfasts, lunches, as refreshing snacks or – and this one is the most exciting – for nutrient-dense desserts.

If you are opting to include more acid-forming foods in your diet, such as meat, grains, caffeine and sweets, it is best to have them earlier in the day, followed by an alkalising smoothie or juice mid-afternoon and a cooked soup in the evening. This will give your body time to rebalance and the food to digest properly before rest. And so, if you have a big brunch planned on the weekend it might be a good idea to have a bowl of alkalising soup for dinner. If you've been out late and have over-indulged then perhaps a cleansing fruit and vegetable smoothie for breakfast might be a good option.

Many leftover vegetable juices and smoothies make great additions to soups which can be enjoyed as part of an evening meal. We also suggest that you vary or alternate the type of ingredients and recipes you use. In addition, you could continue to sip freely on vegetable teas and tisanes as they are a great alternative to caffeinated drinks; drink them warm or chilled as you prefer.

Fitting the cleanse into your life

While it's not our advice to switch to a diet of just smoothies and juices for life, they are a fantastic way to recalibrate your digestive system every couple of months or following those occasions where you might have over-indulged. *The Alkaline Cleanse* is ideal in spring to give your body a break and a fresh start, especially if you are feeling tired and your digestive system sluggish following heavy winter eating.

As mentioned above, the recipes work really well as quick and delicious meal replacements or additions to simple protein sources (like eggs, for example) for the intermittent fasting (5:2) diet as they are low in calories but provide a nutrient-dense meal.

The recipes in the following chapters are sorted into categories based on the main ingredients: Fruits, Greens (fruits and vegetables), Vegetables, Nutri-Boosters (such as seeds and nuts) and Teas and Tisanes. Take a look in your fridge or cupboard, visit the local greengrocers to see what seasonal fruits and vegetables are on offer, and then pick an alkaline drink to improve your day.

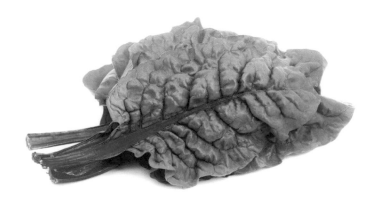

FRUIT JUICES
AND SMOOTHIES

There is no greater luxury than a bowl of fresh fruit but the absolute key to alkaline eating is ripeness. If your fruit is not ripe it is not alkaline. Sadly, too much fruit sold in supermarkets is far from ripe which makes it nutritionally useless. Juicing can help use up less-than-ripe fruit but any nutritional content is devalued, so try to use fruit at its peak.

Glamorous overseas fruit such as peaches, nectarines, papayas and watermelons tend to steal the glory in alkaline eating but home-grown fruits like apples (which are 85 per cent water), pears and plums are excellent bases for juice and come with their own health benefits. Our summer season of brilliant berries is very hard to beat so of course make the most of these when available.

3 plums
¼ purple cabbage
1 beetroot
2 celery stalks
1 orange

AUTUMN PLUM COCKTAIL

Damsons, greengages and Victoria plums offer a wonderful array of colours and flavours that seem to come quickly each week through the autumn. Use whatever variety is in season near you. Imported plums can be a welcome treat in winter but you may need to leave them a while to ripen. Plums are both anti-oxidising and good cleansers of the gut, hence the good digestive reputation of prunes.

Cut the plums in half and remove the stones. Place the flesh in the juicer. Remove the white core from the cabbage and cut the leaves into shreds. Add to the juicer. Peel the beetroot and chop into slices. Add the beetroot and celery to the juicer. Peel the orange and break into segments and add. Mix well and pour into a glass to serve.

1 pear
2 stalks celery
½ cucumber

PEAR, CELERY AND CUCUMBER JUICE

Pears have more pectin (a good fibre) than apples and are easily digested which is one reason why pear is a popular first baby food. Pear skin is valuable in terms of phytonutrients, so leave it on. This is a great way to get celery into your diet.

Cut the pear into quarters (no need to remove the core and pips). Place the pear in the juicer. Add the celery. Peel the cucumber and add. Mix well and pour into a glass to serve.

5 cm slice of
pineapple
½ mango
¼ melon
250 ml coconut
water

TROPICAL STORM

All the tropical fruits have high levels of vitamins A and C and manganese which can be very useful in winter when other ripe fruits are scarce. If you buy the whole fruits store any leftovers in the fridge and use as soon as possible; don't make up a large batch of juice as the vitamins and minerals oxidise quickly.

Peel the pineapple, mango and melon and roughly chop the fruit. Place in a blender, add the coconut water and whizz for one minute until smooth.

1 pear
1 peach
1 green or red
apple
1 lime

PEAR, PEACH AND APPLE JUICE

The peach in this juice adds a comforting thickness, almost like a smoothie, and the lime adds a little edge.

Cut the pear into quarters (no need to remove the core and pips). Place the pear in the juicer. Cut the peach in half and twist out the stone. Cut the apple in half and discard the core and pips. Put the peach and apple in the juicer and juice. Peel the lime and cut into pieces and add to the juicer. If you think you would prefer less lime you could hand-squeeze the lime and add gradually to taste. Mix well and pour into a glass to serve.

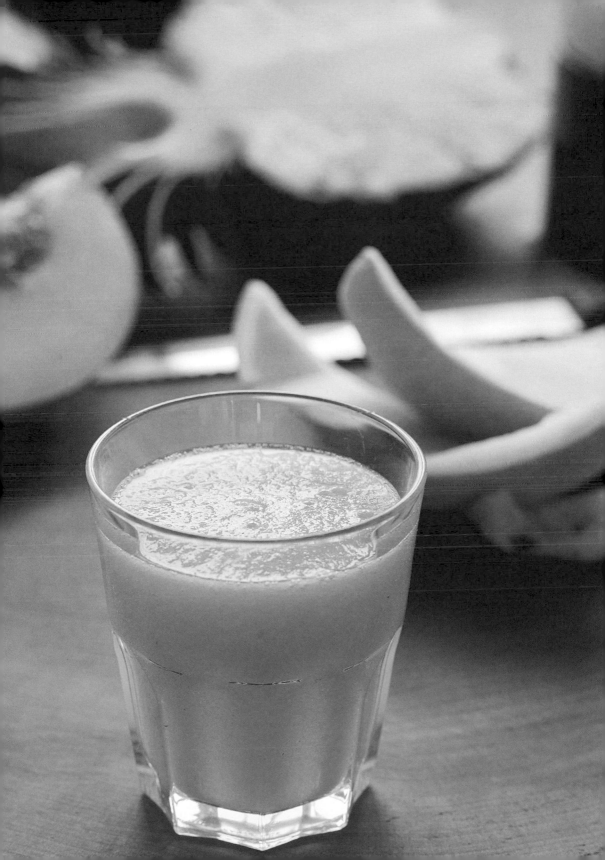

PINK AND GREEN JUICE

1 pink grapefruit
1 green apple
large handful of kale
4 celery stalks
½ cucumber
1 lime

Pink or ruby grapefruits seem to pack more anti-oxidising properties than yellow and have a sweeter flavour. Just half a grapefruit would meet over 60 per cent of your vitamin C daily requirement and 28 per cent of your vitamin A. Pairing it with kale and other good things makes this juice nutrition dynamite.

Peel the grapefruit, divide into segments, and place in the juicer and juice. Cut the apple in half and discard the core and pips. Add the apple. Cut out the stalk of the kale leaves and add the leaves to the juicer. Follow with the celery. Peel the cucumber and add. Peel the lime, cut into chunks, and add to the juicer. Mix well and pour into a glass to serve.

WATERMELON AND CUCUMBER COOLER

large slice of watermelon
2 limes
1 cucumber

TIP: WATERMELON PIPS CAN BE DRIED AND ROASTED AND EATEN AS A SNACK.

Watermelon is a potential companion to any red berry fruit but lime and cucumber are a more unusual match which we love. Watermelon also works well simply juiced on its own; it is a classic cooling summer drink that you can find on beaches all over the world. Keep slices in the fridge so you don't need to add ice before juicing or blending.

Peel the watermelon and cut it into thin slices. Pick out the black seeds as you go but a few in the juice won't matter. Place the watermelon in the juicer and juice. Peel the limes and cucumber and cut into chunks. Add to the juicer. Mix well and pour into a glass to serve.

PASSION FRUIT MOJITO

1 lime
2 passion fruit
1 green apple
250 ml cold filtered water
6 mint leaves
ice cubes, to serve

There is enough flavour in this virgin mojito that you won't miss the rum or sugar. Honest. You can swap the passion fruit for pomegranate seeds for a divine red mojito.

Cut the lime in half and hand-squeeze the juice. Cut the passion fruits in half and scoop out the flesh. Cut the apple in half and discard the core and pips. Place the lime juice, passion fruit and apple in a blender with half the water and whizz for a minute until smooth. Put the mint leaves in your serving glass and muddle (use a muddler, or a wood spoon if you don't have one). Pour the juice over the mint. Add the ice and top with the rest of the water. Use the other end of your muddler or spoon to mix.

MELON AND KIWI CRUSH

¼ melon
2 kiwi fruit
handful of spinach leaves
50 g green grapes
1 teaspoon spirulina powder
125 ml water
ice cubes, to serve

Melons are one of the most easily digestible foods and they are also good sources of vitamin A. Use whichever variety you like. Perhaps surprisingly melons have more beta-carotene than oranges, even the white-fleshed varieties. Melon has fewer polyphenols than other fruits, say, compared to a kiwi, but the amount in this juice still provides an important boost.

Peel the melon and cut into large chunks. Peel the kiwi fruits and cut in half. Place the melon and kiwi fruit in a blender and whizz together until smooth. Add the spinach, grapes, spirulina powder and water and whizz again until smooth. Pour into a glass over ice cubes to serve.

50 g blackberries
50 g blueberries
50 g strawberries
50 g black or red
grapes
125 ml coconut
water
1 lime

BERRY BOOST

All berry fruits juice well but dark-skinned blackberries, blueberries and black grapes pack a little more flavour and contain more anti-oxidising elements than red fruits. Look also for black and red currants in the summer (pick the berries off the stalks) and try red or green gooseberries and tayberries to ring the changes.

Pick over the fruit, discard any discoloured fruit and wash very carefully to remove any bugs or leaves. Place the berries and grapes along with the coconut water in a blender and whizz for one minute until smooth. Cut the lime in half and hand-squeeze the juice. Add as much lime juice as you like to the juice, and pour into a glass to serve.

SHOULD YOU BUY SEEDLESS?

Grape seeds will add extra fibre without altering the flavour of a juice or smoothie too much, so there is no need to buy seedless varieties. And life is definitely too short to de-seed a grape.

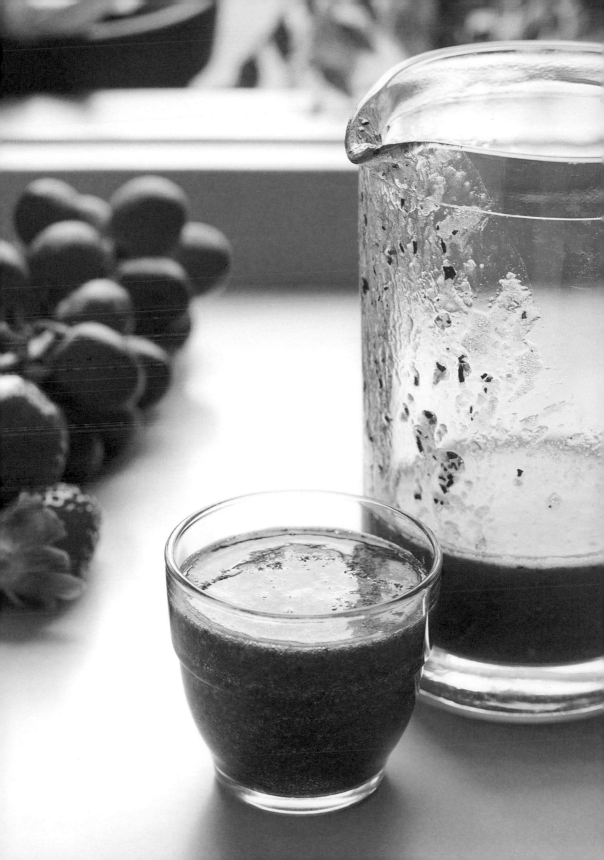

GREEN JUICES
AND SMOOTHIES

There are plenty of modern studies that support the benefits of getting greens into your diet and new juicing technology has made it so much easier. All greens are good for you, and some, such as kale, are really good for you. The darkness of the leaf is usually a good indicator of more minerals and vitamins but even the pale lettuces are a boon. One rich source, which is often overlooked, are the leaves on radishes, turnips and beetroots. They do not keep fresh for very long but if you juice them when you get home you are effectively buying two vegetables for the price of one.

One of the great things about juicing is it transforms vegetables into liquid elixirs and all in less than a minute; it's far quicker than cooking. Extracting the last drops of moisture from your leaves depends on the power of your machinery (see pages 44–46). If you are using a blender then you may find you prefer your juice diluted with water for a less intense brew; from a health perspective the extra fluid is a good thing too.

3 large carrots
1 green apple
handful of parsley

CARROT, APPLE AND PARSLEY JUICE

Carrot and apple juice is a classic combination – the parsley adds a spicy pepperiness and makes it green. Change the flavour and sweetness of the juice by using different apple varieties as they come into season. The difference between a Bramley and a Cox, for example, is night and day. Go easy on the parsley at first; it can be surprisingly potent. Just a handful would supply about five times your daily need for vitamin K.

Top and tail the carrots and add to the juicer. Cut the apple in half, core and discard any pips (there is no need to peel) and add to the juicer. Rough chop the parsley stalks and leaves and feed into the juicer. Mix well.

5 cm slice of
pineapple
3 kale leaves
½ cucumber
½ vanilla pod

PINEAPPLE, KALE AND VANILLA JUICE

This is an unusual combination but the pineapple and kale work well together. You can try this another time using fresh green chilli rather than vanilla if you like.

Slice the skin off the pineapple, remove the hard central core and cut the pineapple into cubes. Add to the juicer. Cut the stalks out of the kale and feed the leaves into the juicer. Peel the cucumber, add to the mixture and juice. Scrape out the seeds from the vanilla pod; you only need a little vanilla to flavour this so add a tiny amount of the seeds and taste as you go, adding more if you like it.

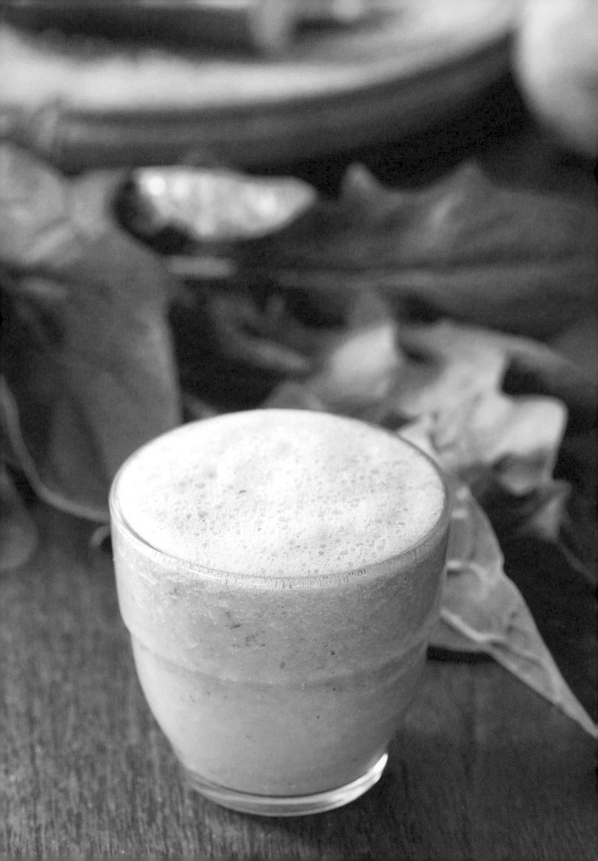

1 courgette
2 pears
¼ fennel
3 broccoli florets
with stalks
handful of spinach

....

TIP: ALWAYS INCLUDE
BROCCOLI STALKS IN
YOUR SMOOTHIES AND
JUICES AS THAT IS
WHERE MOST OF THE
LIQUID IS CONTAINED.

COURGETTE, PEAR
AND FENNEL JUICE

Courgettes get bitter as they age so buy them young and juice as soon as you get back from shopping. Courgettes have few calories but are good sources of vitamin C and potassium. The fennel here gives everything an aniseed twist.

Wash and chop the courgette and add to the juicer. Core the pears (there is no need to peel) and add to the juicer. Cut the fennel vertically so it fits in the juicer easily. Add the broccoli, including the stalks, and the spinach. Mix well and pour into a glass to serve.

1 orange
4 kale leaves
1 kiwi
sprig of mint

....

NOTE: YOU CAN
FIND KIWIS, USUALLY
LABELLED 'GOLDEN
KIWIS', WHICH DO
NOT NEED PEELING
SO YOU CAN JUICE
THEM SKIN AND
ALL. THE FURRY
SKIN IS NUTRITIOUS
AND ADDS FIBRE
BUT IT IS AN
ACQUIRED TASTE.

KIWI, KALE AND MINT JUICE

The flavours here interweave well with each other – this juice is perfect for a late summer afternoon or as a reminder of summer in the winter months.

Peel the orange and add to the juicer. Cut the stalks out of the kale and add the leaves to the juicer. Peel the kiwi and add to the mix. Pick off about 12 mint leaves and add to the juicer. Mix well and pour into a glass to serve.

CORIANDER CRUSH

bunch of coriander
½ cucumber
1 green apple
1 lime

VARIATION: ADD A SMALL HANDFUL OF GREEN OR BLACK GRAPES FOR A CHANGE; THE FLAVOUR ADDS AN ELEGANT TWIST.

Coriander is a wonderful healthy herb; it used to be said it cured smallpox, but modern research points more to its calming effect on the stomach and how it helps lower cholesterol and high blood pressure. This juice makes coriander the star. You might also try the same recipe using fresh basil.

Juice the coriander stalks and leaves. Peel the cucumber and add to the juicer. Cut the apple in half and remove the core and pips. Add to the mix. Peel the lime, cut into chunks, and add to the juicer. Mix well and pour into a glass to serve.

KALE ESPRESSO

5 kale leaves
1 lemon
1 green apple
2 cm ginger root
sprig of mint

NOTE: KALE STALKS TEND TO BE BITTER SO WE SUGGEST CUTTING THEM OUT.

Kale has become fashionable partly because it is the healthiest of the dark leafy greens and it juices so well, but if you have a good supply of Savoy cabbage or spinach they will work well in this recipe too. It is quite an intense, peppery shot, with vitamins A, C and K as well as copper, potassium, iron, manganese and phosphorus. A handful of fresh kale has about 40 calories but packs three grams of protein. The oxalate also means all this goodness is easily absorbed.

Cut the stalks out of the kale and feed the leaves into the juicer. Peel the lemon and discard any pips. Cut the apple in half and discard the core and pips. Add the lemon and apple to the juicer. Peel the ginger and add to the juicer. Pick off about 15 mint leaves and add to the juicer. Mix well and pour into a glass to serve.

½ cabbage or good
handful of kale
leaves
1 green pepper
1 carrot
2 stalks celery
bunch of parsley
12 white grapes

....

NOTE: CABBAGE
LEAVES CAN CLOG
UP YOUR MACHINERY,
SO CUT THE LEAVES
SMALL. THE STALKS
TEND TO BE BITTER,
SO BEST LEAVE THEM
OUT OF THIS JUICE.

CABBAGE OR KALE SOUP JUICE

Filling and nutritious, cabbage or kale is the main ingredient here. You could try a mixture of both, depending on what you have to hand. If you want to make it into a more substantial meal or a longer drink add some chopped tomatoes.

Cut the stalks out of the cabbage or kale and slice the leaves into ribbons. Feed them into the juicer slowly. Cut the pepper into quarters and remove the pith and pips. Add to the juicer. Top and tail the carrot and add to the mix, followed by the celery and the parsley stalks and leaves. Add the grapes and mix well. If you want to make the juice more liquid or sweeter add a few more grapes. Pour into a glass to serve.

1 green apple
2 celery stalks
5 kale leaves
handful watercress
2 cm ginger root
1 lemon

WATERCRESS AND GINGER JUICE

Watercress packs in more vitamins than its fashionable rival rocket, especially when raw. If properly fresh it is really two vegetables in one – the leaves soft like corn salad, the stems crunchy as bean sprouts. Here you get the best of both.

Cut the apple into chunks and discard the core. Juice. Add the celery stalks. Cut out the kale stalks and feed into the mix, then add the watercress. Peel the ginger and add. Lastly, peel and add the lemon, or just cut in half and squeeze into the mix. Stir.

1 green apple
3 celery stalks
½ cucumber
2 cm ginger root
2 kale leaves
1 lemon

....

NOTE: CUCUMBER SKIN
CONTAINS SILICA WHICH
IS A VITAL COMPONENT
FOR HEALTHY TISSUES
SO YOU MIGHT PREFER
TO LEAVE IT ON, BUT
THE FLAVOUR IS QUITE
HARSH. IF YOU WANT
TO INCLUDE THE SKIN,
IT IS BETTER TO BUY
ORGANIC CUCUMBER.

EVERYDAY GREEN TONIC

A crisp green apple combined with ginger makes this a refreshing tonic that can give you a lift at any time of the day. It is an easy way to get some kale into your diet too.

Cut the apple in half and remove the core and pips. Add to the juicer followed by the celery. Peel the cucumber and cut into thin lengths and juice. Peel the ginger root and add. Cut the stalks out of the kale and feed the leaves into the juicer. Peel the lemon, discard any pips, and add to the juicer. Stir well and pour into a glass to serve.

½ avocado
1 small banana
2 kiwi fruit
2 limes
handful of watercress
375 ml coconut water

KIWI AND AVOCADO SMOOTHIE

Good enough for dessert this has a lovely creamy texture and is sweetened by the kiwi fruit and coconut. Watercress is very peppery so add as much as you like, tasting as you go.

Peel the avocado, banana, kiwi fruits and limes and discard any pips. Place all the ingredients in a blender and whizz for one minute until smooth. Add the watercress and mix well; you might like to add a little watercress at a time and taste as you go. Pour into a glass to serve.

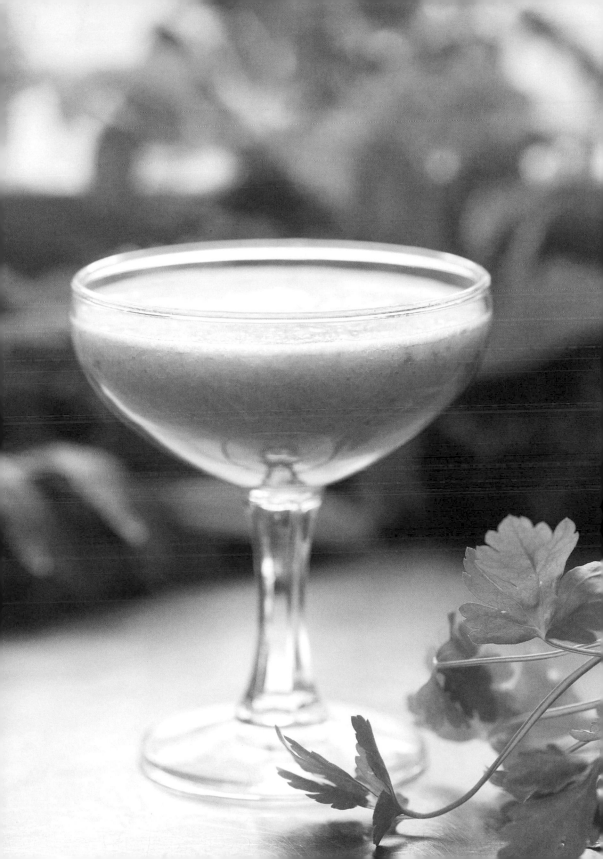

VEGETABLE JUICES AND SMOOTHIES

....

Humble root vegetables are among the richest sources of alkalising minerals in the garden. If you can use organic then there is no need to peel, especially if they are young and tender. Not every vegetable is easy to juice; leeks for example, are alkaline, but they can wreak havoc with your juicer so we use them cooked in soups instead.

Carrots are the kings of the juicedom, either juiced on their own or mixed in equal parts with other vegetables or fruits – celery and pear work well. Carrots also love ginger. Beetroots give a glorious colour and their leaves, when young, are excellent for juicing. Celery is an essential juicing ingredient and can be added to many recipes. Sweet potatoes juice very well and are easier to digest than white potatoes.

6 carrots
1 apple
½ celery

CARROT, APPLE AND CELERY JUICE

Carrot juice might be the single most persuasive reason to upgrade your blender to a proper juicer. You can turn carrots into juices so quickly but most blenders will struggle. Carrot works with so many other ingredients especially orange, coriander, ginger and pepper; this is a delicious combination.

Top and tail the carrots and juice. Cut the apple in half and discard the core and pips. Add to the juicer. Cut the celery lengthwise and feed into the juicer. Mix well and pour into a glass to serve.

1 fennel bulb
¼ celeriac
1 parsnip
1 carrot
200 g green grapes

....

NOTE: FENNEL IS A GREAT ANTI-INFLAMMATORY. THE BULB HAS A MILDER TASTE THAN THE FRONDS AND BOTH ARE SUITABLE FOR USING IN JUICES.

FENNEL AND CELERIAC MINERAL BOOST

The root vegetables you might be more used to finding alongside a roast lunch or in a soup can be a welcome surprise in a juice. The grapes here add a wine-like quality.

Roughly chop the fennel bulb and fronds. Cut the sides of the celeriac away so you are left with a clean white cube, then trim into manageable lengths. Top and tail the parsnip and carrot, and peel if necessary. Put everything through the juicer, with the grapes last. Mix well and pour into a glass to serve.

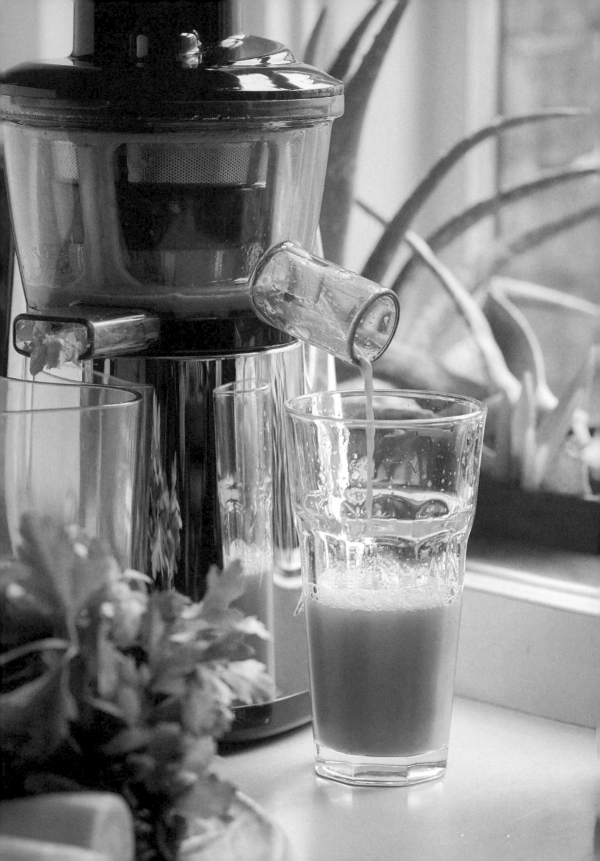

SAUERKRAUT SHOTS

2 carrots
100 g sauerkraut
5 sprigs parsley
ice cubes or cold
water, to serve

Sauerkraut produces lactic acid and live enzyme cultures that give cabbage a pleasing sour tang. It is one of the most potent plant-based sources of gut-friendly probiotics. Look for sauerkraut that does not have vinegar or wine added as they inhibit the growth of the beneficial bacteria.

Trim and peel the carrots. Place all the ingredients, including the parsley stalks, in a blender and whizz for one minute until smooth. Pour into a glass and add a few ice cubes or a few drops of cold water to dilute to your taste.

BEETROOT DAY-AFTER JUICE

1 beetroot
1 parsnip
2 carrots
1 apple
2 celery stalks
2 cm ginger root
small handful of
parsley
½ tablespoon
linseed, pumpkin,
avocado or olive oil

NOTE: OILS LIKE
LINSEED, PUMPKIN,
AVOCADO AND OLIVE
CONTAIN FAT-SOLUBLE
VITAMINS A, D, E AND
K; EATING THEM AS
PART OF A JUICE OR
SMOOTHIE HELPS THOSE
NUTRIENTS BECOME
MORE EASILY ABSORBED
INTO THE BODY.

Beetroot has blood-cleansing properties so is perfect as a pick-me-up after a big night out. Ginger is great for digestion, celery is anti-inflammatory and antioxidant-rich, and the carrots and apple provide sweetness as well as vitamin A and C. You can choose whichever oil you have to hand; they each have their own benefits.

Peel and cut the beetroot, parsnip and carrots into large chunks. Cut the apple in half and discard the core and pips. Cut the apple and celery into large chunks. Put all the ingredients, except the oil, though the juicer. Add the oil and mix well. Pour into a glass to serve.

LETTUCE AND BERRY SLUSHIE

4 romaine lettuce leaves
½ small cucumber
2 celery stalks
75 g mixed berries such as strawberries, raspberries and blackberries
125 ml cold water

A perfect alternative to those ready-made drinks laden with sugar and artificial colours and flavours, this slushie is made with delicious crisp lettuce and summer berries. Look for very ripe berries; buy more than you need and freeze for a ready supply. You can blend fruit straight from the freezer; otherwise, you might like to add some ice.

Put the romaine lettuce leaves in the blender. Peel the cucumber and chop into chunks, then add to the blender. Slice the celery into chunks and add. Pick over the berries and discard anything discoloured. Add the berries and water and whizz for a minute until smooth. Pour into a glass to serve.

PURPLE HAZE

¼ small red cabbage
1 small fennel bulb
200 g black or red grapes
1 lemon, to serve

The wonderful aniseed flavour of fennel combines really well with the sweetness of black or red grapes. The red cabbage is anti-bacterial and lends a regal purple colour.

Remove the white core from the red cabbage and cut the cabbage into chunks, across the leaves. Place in the juicer and juice. Cut the fennel into quarters and add to the juicer, followed by the grapes. Finish with a generous squeeze of lemon juice to taste. Mix well and pour into a glass to serve.

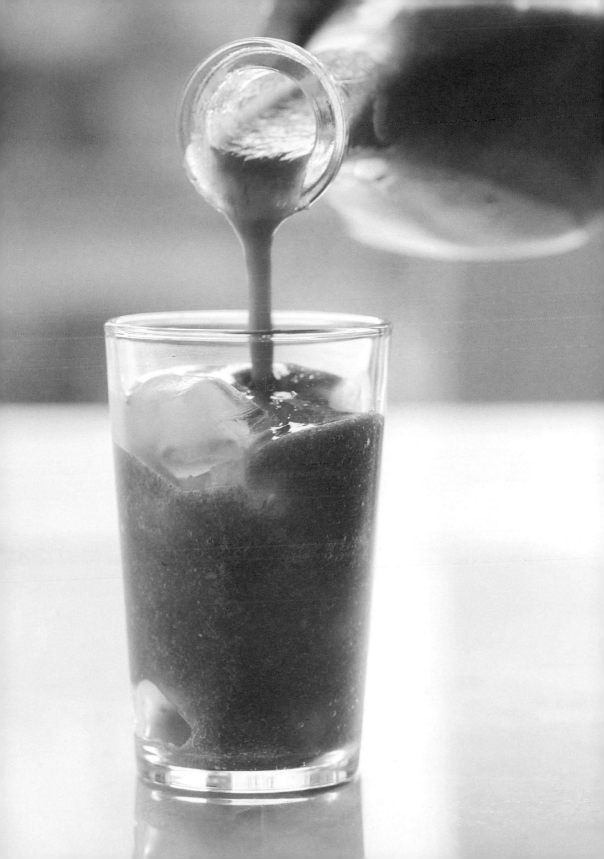

1 red pepper
bunch of red grapes
handful of spinach
leaves
1 green or red apple

RED PEPPER PUNCH

One red pepper provides three times the daily recommended amount of vitamin C and all the vitamin A; that's even better than an orange. Red peppers have twice the vitamin C of younger green peppers. They can be mixed happily with carrots and oranges without adding a strong flavour, or you can juice them for a shot on their own.

Cut the pepper in half and remove the pips and white pith. Cut the pepper into lengths and feed into the juicer. Remove the grapes from the stalk and add as many as you like; about the same amount as the pepper is a good balance. Add the spinach leaves. Cut the apple in half and discard the core and pips. Add to the juicer. Mix well and pour into a glass to serve.

1 small sweet potato
2 carrots
2 oranges

SWEET POTATO SMOOTHIE

Sweet potato lends a surprising creaminess to juices and smoothies. It is also supremely alkaline. White potato varieties tend to create gas and wind so we don't usually eat them raw or juice them.

Peel the sweet potato and cut into chunks. Place in the juicer, and juice. Top and tail the carrots and add them to the juicer. Peel the oranges and break into segments and add to the juicer. Mix well and pour into a glass to serve.

2 large
ripe tomatoes
1 small red chilli
1 small green apple
3 celery stalks
1 lemon
sea or rock salt and
pepper, to taste
ice cubes, to serve

VIRGIN MARY

Home-made juices are always better than buying commercially made ones and they are usually much cheaper. You can also make them exactly to your taste; add as much or as little chilli as you like to this. Chilli revs up your digestion and even a little can be enough to make you sweat, which is one of the body's ways to eliminate toxins.

Cut the tomatoes into quarters and place in the juicer. Cut open the chilli and discard the seeds. Cut the apple in half and discard the core and pips. Add to the juicer. Juice two of the celery stalks. Add a good squeeze of lemon juice, a pinch of salt and a grind of fresh pepper. Pour into a glass over ice cubes. Use the remaining celery stalk as a garnish, and to stir the mixture together.

CHILLI POWER

The larger the chilli, usually the less heat it has. Removing the seeds removes some of the heat too. Chillies are alkaline and full of good things, plus they add zip to lots of recipes. When preparing chillies wear gloves as they can burn your fingers, and avoid touching your eyes.

NUTRI-BOOST RECIPES

These recipes give you easy ways to add nutrient-packed extras to your diet such as chia seeds, hemp seeds, pumpkin seeds and cardamom – all things we know are good for the body.

The great thing about smoothies and juices is you can add literally anything you wish, even things that you might not like very much but you know might be good for you. You can add a little celery or spinach into a juice and hide the flavour but get all the benefits. You can be your own modern-day herbalist.

Some of these ingredients might be new to you but your body is a great guide to what you need and might have been missing nutritionally. Almond milk, for example, can readily replace cow's milk. Equally, watermelon juice can make a welcome change from citrus. If you have a craving for cardamom, then it might be that your body is asking you for it, or if you have a natural disliking of figs then don't force yourself to eat them. The point is to be in tune with yourself. Experiment and see what you like the sound of and how you feel after trying one of these booster recipes.

PUMPKIN SEED SMOOTHIE

150 g pumpkin
1 cm cinnamon bark
1 tablespoon pumpkin seeds
1 teaspoon chia seeds
1 teaspoon hemp seeds
125 ml almond or coconut milk

Pumpkin is a satisfying and sweet source of vitamin A. Eating it with pumpkin seeds and hemp seeds helps your body to absorb its vitamin A. Pumpkin seeds are brilliant to eat as they help promote a healthy digestive system, and the hemp seeds are the only plant-based source of the complete spectrum of amino acids. For maximum nutrition use pumpkin raw, but if the taste is too strong for you, steam it for 15 minutes first.

Peel the pumpkin and set the seeds to one side. Cut the pumpkin into chunks. Using a grinder or a pestle and mortar crush the cinnamon and the seeds (including the seeds from the pumpkin) together. Put the pumpkin and seed mixture into a blender and add the almond or coconut milk. Whizz for a minute until smooth. Pour into a glass to serve.

CREAMY CHAI MILK

10 Brazil nuts
10 almonds
1 cm cinnamon bark
2 cardamom cloves
1 clove
1 tablespoon honey
250 ml almond milk

Brazil nuts are an excellent source of selenium, essential to healthy thyroid function. When blended, they make a creamy, textured milk. Fragrant spices add warming, tea-like comfort.

Using a grinder or a pestle and mortar, crush the Brazil nuts, almonds, cinnamon, cardamom and clove into a fine powder. Transfer to a blender and add the honey and almond milk. Whizz for a minute until smooth. Pour into a glass to serve.

1 young coconut or ½ litre coconut milk
1 small red or green chilli
1 cm vanilla pod
1 cardamom seed
2–3 tablespoons raw cacao powder
sea or rock salt

AZTEC CHOCOLATE DRINK

Many iced chocolate drinks are loaded with sugar and additives. You can make your own delicious, creamy, iced chocolate drink using the water and flesh of a young coconut (you can use coconut milk but it won't have the same texture). Raw cacao adds the chocolate hit and a little chilli, cardamom and sea or rock salt lift the whole thing into something special.

If you are using a fresh coconut, cut it open (see below), catching all the milk. Scrape out the coconut flesh. Put the coconut flesh and milk (or coconut milk, if using) into a blender. Cut open the chilli and scrape out and discard the seeds. Crush lightly with the back of a knife and add as much as you like to the blender (you can always add more at the end). Cut open and crush the vanilla pod and add to the blender. Bash the cardamom seed with a wooden spoon to release the oils. Put the cardomom seed and cacao powder into the blender and whizz everything for a minute until smooth. Add a little salt to taste. Pour into a glass or milk bottle to serve.

HOW TO OPEN A COCONUT

Young drinking coconuts are full of creamy, soft flesh that can be scooped out and turned into delicious smoothies. To open a coconut use a serrated knife to cut off the top, about three centimetres down, then pour out the milk. You could also use a screwdriver or skewer to make a hole either side and pour out the milk before cutting the coconut in half and scooping out the flesh.

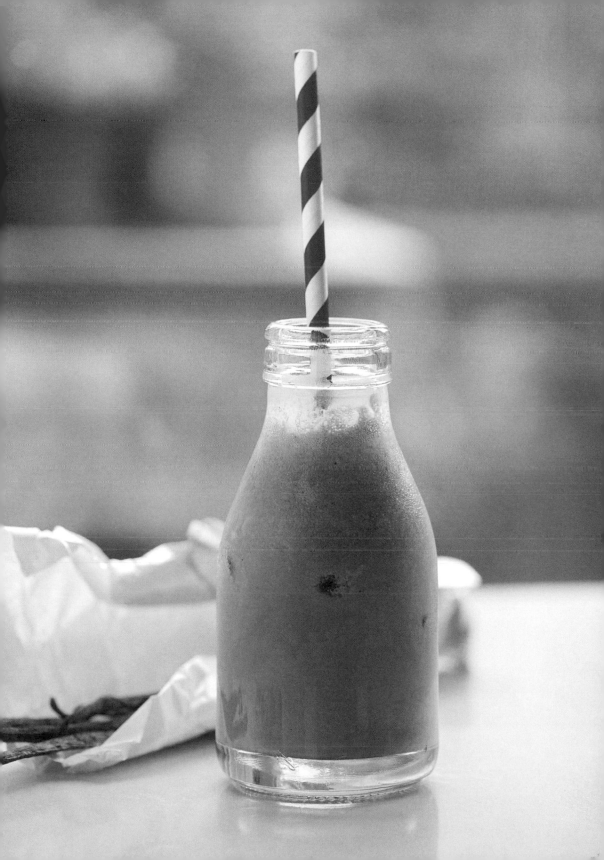

BANANA, DATE AND NUT SHAKE

1 banana
3 Medjool dates
10 almonds, skin on
1 tablespoon sunflower seeds
1 tablespoon flaxseeds
200 ml almond milk

This tastes of chocolate and caramel so you might think it is not good for you, but in a miraculous way it is. Packed with seeds and nuts this is a meal in itself.

Peel the banana and pit the dates. Put the banana, dates, almonds, seeds and almond milk in a blender and whizz for one minute until smooth. Pour into a glass to serve.

APPLE AND OAT OVERNIGHT SMOOTHIE

1 green apple
50 g rolled oats
1 tablespoon flaxseeds
6 almonds, skin on
125 ml almond milk

Prepare this the night before so it is ready to eat in the morning; soaking the oats in apple juice means that you don't have to cook them, making this a very quick breakfast. Freshly juiced apples have more fibre and less sugar than most commercial apple juices that are usually made from nutrient-devoid reconstituted blends.

Cut the apple in half and discard the core and pips. Put into a juicer and juice. Put the oats, flaxseeds and almonds in a bowl and pour the apple juice over. Leave to soak overnight. In the morning, add the almond milk. Pour into a blender and whizz until smooth. Pour into a glass to serve.

100 g mixed nuts such as almonds, Brazil nuts and walnuts
2 tablespoons mixed seeds such as sunflower, pumpkin and flax seeds
1 cm ginger root
75 g rolled oats
1 tablespoon honey
1 tablespoon raw cacao powder
250 ml almond milk

CHOCOLATE AND NUT WHIP

Oats, raw cacao and ginger give this whip a lovely biscuit texture, a little like cookie dough. If you are craving tea and biscuits try this nutrient-packed alternative which will help control blood sugar levels. You could eat this for breakfast too.

Using a grinder or a pestle and mortar crush the nuts and seeds until cracked open. Put them in the blender. Peel and grate the ginger and add to the blender. Add the oats, honey, cacao powder and almond milk and whizz for a minute until blended. Pour into a glass to serve.

SUPER RAW CACAO

Raw cacao powder retains the living enzymes of the cocoa plant and is rich in magnesium, phosphorus, iron, potassium, calcium, zinc, copper and manganese. You need only a little as it is strong-flavoured. Do not use commerical chocolate powders instead as they will have lost the enzymes during processing and are often mixed with sugar.

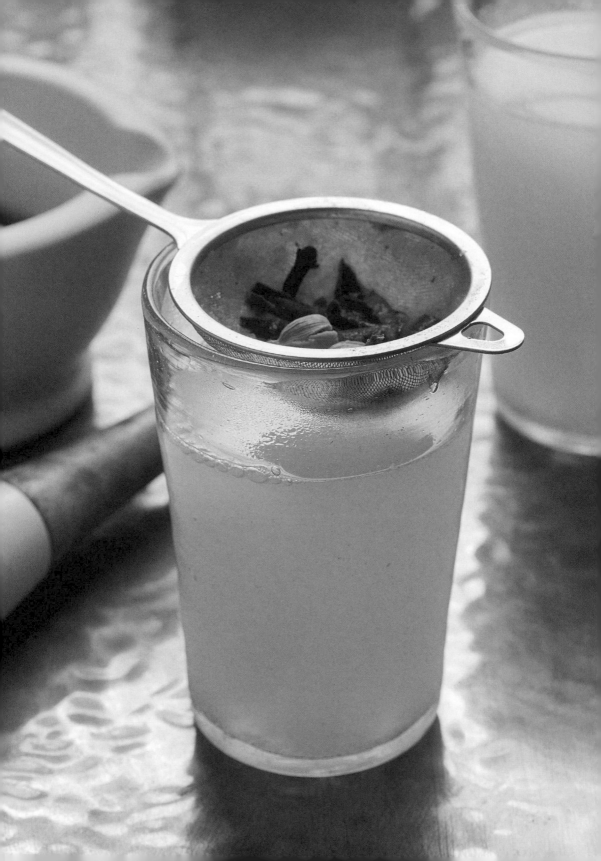

APPLE AND GINGER CORDIAL

2 cm ginger root
1 green or red apple
1 pear
1 cardamom seed
1 clove
1 cm cinnamon bark
100 ml hot water
1 teaspoon honey

A versatile, vitamin-packed drink that you can sip on its own over ice cubes, or diluted with a little ice cold water. It is also a great alternative to tea and coffee – just top up with hot water; the spices and ginger add to the warming effect.

Peel the ginger and juice. Cut the apple and pear in half and discard the cores and pips. Add to the juicer. Using a pestle and mortar or a wooden spoon and a bowl, crush the cardamom seed, clove and cinnamon lightly to release their oils. Put them in a bowl and pour over the hot water. Add the juice from the fruit and ginger. Leave to infuse for 5 minutes. Strain, then add the honey. Mix well and pour into a glass or cup. Top up with cold or hot water if you like.

CAROTENOID COCKTAIL

1 sweet potato
20 g kale leaves
2 tomatoes
1 teaspoon spirulina

Research has shown that this mix provides some surprising results – notably raising immunity levels. Note that the darker the skin of the sweet potato, and the riper your tomatoes, the more carotenoids and vitamins your juice will contain. This is also an easy recipe for adding spirulina to your diet.

Cut the sweet potato into chunks, place in the juicer, and juice. Cut out the stalks from the kale and feed the leaves into the juicer. Cut the tomatoes into quarters and juice. Add the spirulina and mix well before pouring into a glass to serve.

TEAS AND TISANES

We tend to overlook the power of herbs; herb teas and tisanes were our original juices and were everyday medicine in the Middle Ages. Just try a cup of lemon balm or chamomile tea before going to sleep to experience their calming properties.

Buying fresh, good-quality herbs is fairly easy now, but if you can grow your own it can work out much cheaper and you only pick what you need. Packaged teas can be very expensive, with the box packaging often having more vitality than the tea inside. If you use fresh leaves or dry your own you know how fresh they are; some boxes of tea can be months old.

Making herb tea is no different from making tea with anything else; you just need a cup, hot (not quite boiling) water, a few minutes to let the leaves impart their goodness, and a tea strainer. As a rough guide a small handful of fresh leaves makes about two teaspoons of dried leaves. You need about one teaspoon to make tea for one person.

We use herb teas as a base for juices and smoothies too, and you can use them when a recipe calls for water. It is a good way of getting the benefits of the herbs into your diet.

The teas here have been organised so that those best to drink in the morning come first, and those perfect for an evening cup are towards the end of the section.

6 fresh or
1 teaspoon of dried
sage leaves
200 ml hot, almost
boiling water

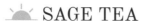 SAGE TEA

*Old herbal remedy books list many benefits of sage, including
helping digestion and treating the menopause. It may also
help with Alzheimer's disease. You can use the tea to fight off
infection, either by drinking it or using it to clean wounds. It is
not a good idea to drink sage tea if you are pregnant or have
just had a baby because it can affect your milk supply.*

Put the sage leaves in a cup and pour over the hot water (or
place the leaves in a sealed tea infuser). Leave to infuse for
three or four minutes. Strain out the sage before drinking.

2 cm ginger root
200 ml hot, almost
boiling water
a few drops of fresh
lemon juice

 GINGER TEA

*Warming ginger has been used in Eastern herbal teas against
nausea and travel sickness and to make a sweat to break
a fever. Many juice bars use ginger to give their fruit and
vegetable drinks a kick – think of the classic combination of
carrot and ginger – but ginger can be a star on its own. If the
taste is too strong for you, soothe it down with a teaspoon of
honey or molasses.*

Peel the ginger and grate it into your cup. Pour the water over
the ginger and leave to infuse for five minutes. Squeeze over a
few drops of lemon juice to serve.

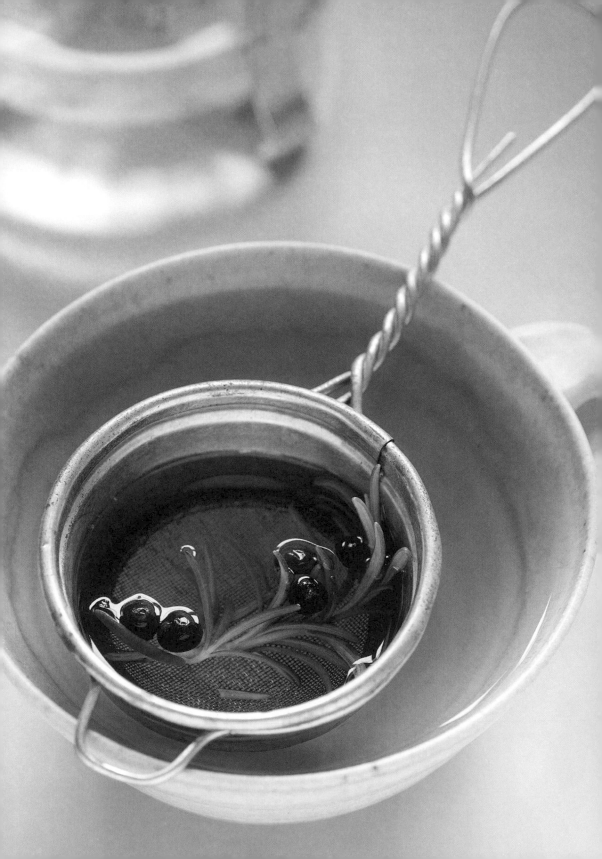

1 sprig of fresh or
1 teaspoon
of dried rosemary
4 juniper berries
200 ml hot, almost
boiling water

 ## ROSEMARY AND JUNIPER TEA

Rosemary is thought to stimulate the mind and calm the stomach. It is a good source of iron, calcium and vitamin B6. Juniper berries are not actually berries, but tiny pine cones, and they are full of antioxidants; they pep up this infusion in a unique way.

Put the rosemary and juniper berries in a cup and pour over the hot water. Leave to infuse for three or four minutes (if you leave it any longer the tea can become quite bitter). Strain out the rosemary and berries before drinking.

3–4 raspberry
leaves
200 ml hot, almost
boiling water
1 teaspoon
echinacea liquid
1 raspberry

 ## ECHINACEA AND RASPBERRY LEAF TEA

Echinacea stimulates the body's immune system to fight off bacterial and viral attacks and is a popular remedy for 'flu and colds. The medicinal properties are found in the leaves, purple flowers and roots and they are made into widely available liquids. Native to North America, echinacea was used for medicinal purposes by Plains Indians and it was on the USA list of official approved therapies until 1950 when it was replaced by antibiotics. If you grow raspberries pick a few leaves to add to this tea or buy the dried ones.

Put the raspberry leaves in a cup and pour over the hot water. Leave to infuse for five minutes. Add the echinacea and stir in. Strain out the leaves and serve with the fresh raspberry on top.

1 lime
10 fresh mint leaves
ice cubes and
sparkling mineral
water, to serve
1 sprig mint, to
serve

 # MINT AND LIME ICED TEA

There are many varieties of mint from peppermint to pineapple mint but it is Moroccan mint that is traditionally used in tea. It encourages a light sweating and has been used traditionally to combat fever and congestion as well as to cool in hot temperatures. You can serve mint drinks hot, or as here, chilled as a refreshing summer drink.

Cut the lime into wedges and place in a bowl or mortar with the mint leaves. Using a pestle, muddler or wooden spoon crush to release their aromatic oils. Put a few ice cubes in a glass or bottle and add the crushed lime and mint leaves. Top up with sparkling mineral water and stir well.

1 stalk lemongrass
200 ml hot, almost
boiling water
stevia leaves or
agave syrup

....

NOTE: TRY MIXING AN
UNSWEETENED VERSION
OF THIS ICED TEA WITH
THE JUICE OF ONE RED
PEPPER, TWO CARROTS
AND A FEW SPRIGS OF
CORIANDER FOR AN
ASIAN-STYLE CARROT
REFRESHER.

 # LEMONGRASS ICED TEA

This tea is best if you use fresh lemongrass; the trick is to find truly fresh sticks. Lemongrass should be green and pliant, not dried out and crackly. It can grow in a sheltered window box so it is possible to have a fresh supply all the year round. It also combines well with coconut water for juicing and, of course, for use in Thai recipes. Lemongrass is excellent for digestion, to calm nerves and to stimulate and purify the blood.

Crush the lemongrass in a cup using the end of a wooden spoon (use a pestle and mortar if you prefer) to release the oils. Pour over the hot water and leave to steep for five minutes. Stir in a little agave syrup or a crushed stevia leaf, strain and leave to cool. Serve over ice.

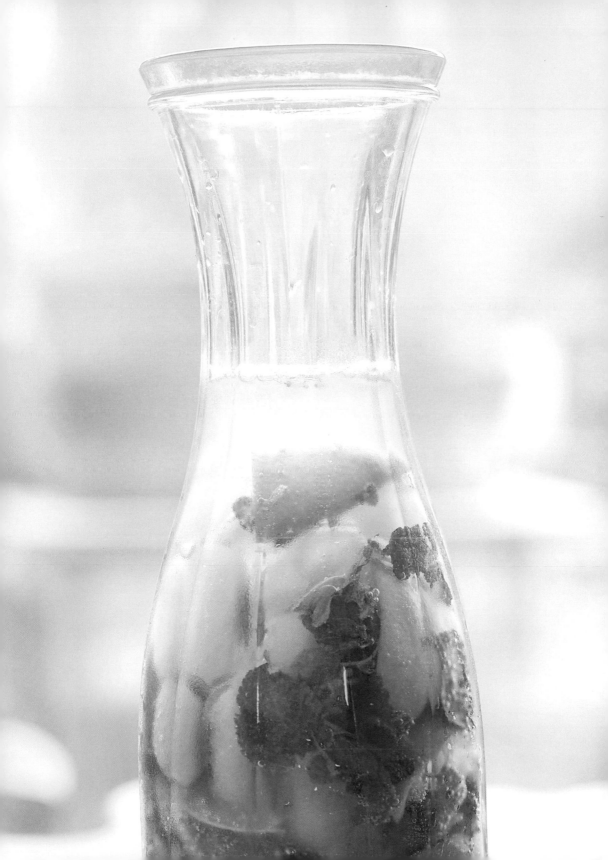

2 teaspoons dried
blackberry leaves
200 ml hot, almost
boiling water

 # BLACKBERRY LEAF TEA

Next time you go blackberry picking, pick some leaves to dry at home. Herbalists use blackberry leaves as a source of vitamin C and tannins, which are good for the immune system.

Put the blackberry leaves in a cup and pour over the hot water (or place the leaves in a sealed tea infuser). Leave to infuse for five minutes. Strain the leaves out before drinking.

3 rose hips
1 fruit berry tea bag
200 ml hot, almost
boiling water

....

NOTE: YOU CAN USE
ROSE HIPS FROM
YOUR GARDEN BUT
THIS IS NOT A GOOD
IDEA IF THE ROSE
PLANTS HAVE BEEN
FED OR SPRAYED
WITH CHEMICALS.

 # ROSE HIP AND FRUIT BERRY TEA

Rose hips are the seed pods at the base of the rose blossom. They contain vitamin C, calcium, iron, selenium and zinc so are well worth using in tea. On their own they make a sharp tea so here we combine them with fruit tea to add sweetness.

Put the rose hips in a cup and pour over the hot water. Leave to infuse for five minutes. Add the tea bag and steep for another minute or two. Remove the rose hips and tea bag before drinking.

1 teaspoon dried
chamomile leaves
and flowers
250 ml hot, almost
boiling water

 # CHAMOMILE TEA

The medicinal value of this tea is mainly in the flowers. It is a great drink for bedtime as the chamomile has a calming effect. It takes a little longer to brew than other teas, about six or seven minutes. You can grow chamomile from seed.

Place the leaves and flowers in a cup and pour over the hot water (or place the leaves in a sealed tea infuser). Leave to infuse for six to seven minutes. Strain out the leaves and flowers before drinking.

1 tablespoon dried
lemon balm leaves
1 teaspoon dried
angelica root
1 lemon
nutmeg
2 coriander seeds
200 ml hot, almost
boiling water

CARMELITE WATER

*This ancient remedy can be traced back to French Carmelite
nuns in 1611. It was used as a therapeutic tea and sometimes
to infuse wine and vodka; it was thought to reduce anxiety and
aid restful sleep. The key ingredient is lemon balm, also known
as Melissa or bee balm. Angelica has similar properties and
both are used in this tisane, which can be served hot or cold.*

Mix the lemon balm leaves and angelica root together in a cup.
Cut a strip of lemon peel from the lemon and add. Grate a little
of the nutmeg over. Crush the coriander seeds with a pestle
and mortar and add to the mix. Pour over the hot water and
steep for two or three minutes. Strain and serve.

1 tablespoon cloves
200 ml hot, almost
boiling water

CLOVE TEA

*Cloves are often used to flavour fruit punches, but they can
also have a starring role on their own. To get the antioxidant
flavonoids, vitamin C, manganese, magnesium and omega-3
fatty acids from cloves you need to use really fresh cloves. You
can test how fresh they are before buying by pressing with your
thumbnail to see if there is any of the oil left.*

Crush the cloves with a pestle and mortar or in a grinder;
aim for small pieces rather than a powder. Put into a cup and
pour over the hot water. Leave to infuse for 10–20 minutes,
depending on how strong you like the tea. Add more hot water
if you like.

ACKNOWLEDGEMENTS

Dr Stephan Domenig

I would like to say thank you to Drew Smith, Silvia Langford and the Elwin Street team for their endless support, to all my patients who have helped me learn; and, last but not least, to my wife and my children for all of their support and love.

Martyna Angell

I would like to thank Dr Domenig for his inspiring vision and the team at Elwin Street – Silvia Langford, Julie Takasaki and Lucy Kingett in particular, for the opportunity they have given me to develop recipes for this book and to share the same passion for real whole food I try to encourage my blog reader towards, here. I also wanted to thank Drew Smith for his support and knowledgeable feedback. To my family, a big thank you for inspiring me toward healthier living and catering the same way for you, every day.

Modern Books would like to thank everyone at the FX Mayr Health Center for their help in creating this book, Drew Smith, Nicola Collings, Becky Alexander and Joe Woodhouse.

Modern Books would also like to thank the following for kindly lending the equipment listed:

The Omega Vert VSJ 843R Juicer available from UK Juicers
The Viva Collection HR1863/01 Juicer from Philips Consumer Lifestyle UK
The Juice Fountain Max from Breville

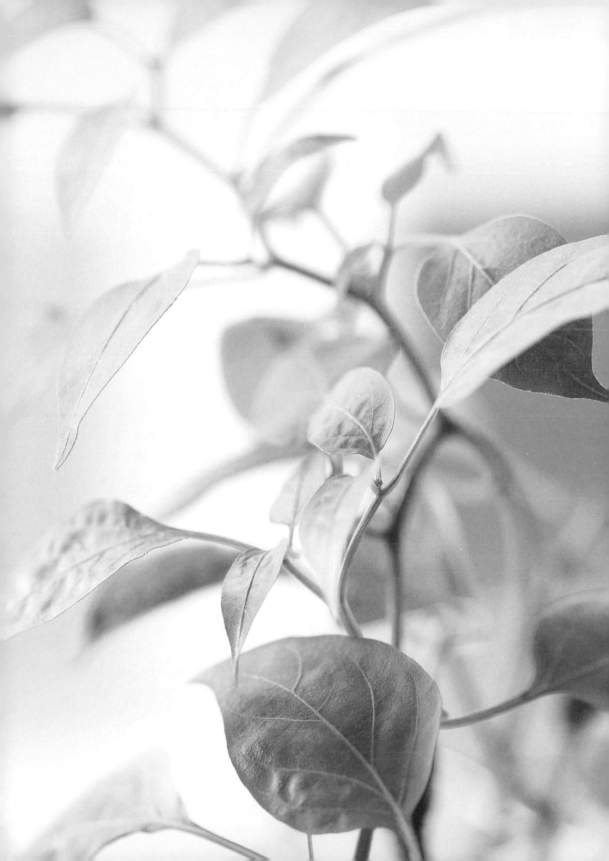

RECIPE FINDER

INDEX

First published in Great Britain in 2015
By Modern Books
An imprint of Elwin Street Limited
3 Percy Street
London W1T 1DE
www.elwinstreet.com

ISBN 978-1-906761-63-9
6 7 8 9 10   5 4 3 2 1

Disclaimer: The advice and recipes in this book are intended as a personal guide to healthy living. However, this information is not intended to provide medical advice and it should not replace the guidance of a qualified physician or other healthcare professional. Decisions about your health should be made by you and your healthcare provider based on the specific circumstances of your health, risk factors, family history and other considerations. See your healthcare provider before making major dietary changes or embarking on an exercise programme, especially if you have existing health problems, medical conditions or chronic diseases. The author and publishers have made every effort to ensure that the information in this book is safe and accurate, but they cannot accept liability for any resulting injury or loss or damage to either property or person, whether direct or consequential and howsoever arising.

Photo Credits

Alessandra Spairani: 35. Drew Smith: 17. FX Mayr Health Center: 10. Getty Images: 45 (Alexandra Grablewski). Joe Woodhouse: 1, 2, 3, 4, 7, 8, 12, 26, 25, 27, 28, 29, 30, 31, 32, 38, 41, 45, 48, 52, 55, 61, 64, 67, 70, 73, 79, 82, 86, 90, 93, 94, 101, 104, 108, 113, 116, 119, 125, 128, 132, 135, 141. Martyna Angell: 11, 45. Shutterstock: Throughout (Alex Illi), 32 (iomis, gephoto), 37 (rng), 53 (Ian 2010, Sommai), 58 (maxpro), 59 (Egor Rodychenko, Alexlukin), 65 (domnitsky, Swapan Photography), 71 (Kostiantyn Fastov, Zorandim), 76 (Arina P Habich), 77 (margouillat photo, Nattika), 83 (Viktor Kunz, Jiang Hongyan), 88 (Charlotte Lake), 89 (Karchenko Ruslan, Nattika), 97 (Jovan Nikolic)

Printed in China